Health Needs of Women as They Age

About the Editors

Sharon Golub is a professor of psychology at the College of New Rochelle and adjunct professor of psychiatry at New York Medical College. As a clinician, teacher, and researcher, she has a long standing interest in women's physical and psychological well-being. Dr. Golub is the editor of three other books, *Menarche, Lifting the Curse of Menstruation,* and *Health Care of the Female Adolescent;* and she has contributed many papers to scientific journals. She is currently editor of *Women & Health.*

Rita Jackaway Freedman is a clinical psychologist and consultant at the Center for Behavioral Psychology, White Plains, NY. Formerly a professor of psychology and women's studies, she has published numerous papers in the area of gender differences and the psychology of women. Dr. Freedman is currently completing a book on the influence of beauty in women's lives and serves as associate editor of *Women & Health.*

Health Needs of Women as They Age

Edited by
Sharon Golub
Rita Jackaway Freedman

Health Needs of Women as They Age was originally published in 1985 by The Haworth Press, Inc. It has also been published as *Women & Health,* Volume 10, Numbers 2/3, Summer/Fall 1985.

Harrington Park Press
New York • Binghamton

ISBN 0-918393-23-X

Published by

Harrington Park Press, Inc.
28 East 22 Street
New York, NY 10010

Harrington Park Press, Inc., is a subsidiary of The Haworth Press, Inc., 28 East 22 Street, New York, New York 10010.

Health Needs of Women as They Age was originally published in 1985 by The Haworth Press, Inc. It has also been published as *Women & Health,* Volume 10, Numbers 2/3, Summer/Fall 1985.

Library of Congress Cataloging in Publication Data
Main entry under title:

Health needs of women as they age.

    Reprint. Originally published: New York : Haworth Press, c1985.
    Includes bibliographies.
    1. Aged women—Health and hygiene—Addresses, essays, lectures. 2. Aged women—Diseases—Addresses, essays, lectures. 3. Aged women—Medical care—Addresses, essays, lectures. 4. Aging—Addresses, essays, lectures. I. Golub, Sharon. II. Freedman, Rita Jackaway.
[RA564.85.H43 1985b]   362.1'088042   85-7642
ISBN 0-918393-23-X

CONTENTS

Contributors

Myrna Lewis, ACSW
Instructor
Department of Community Medicine
Mount Sinai School of Medicine
City University of New York
One Gustave Levy Place
New York, NY 10029

Eloise Rathbone-McCuan, PhD
Director, Social Work Program
University of Vermont
499 C Waterman
Burlington, VT 05405

Dulcy B. Miller, MS
Assistant Clinical Professor of Community Health
Albert Einstein College of Medicine
Administrative Director
The Nathan Miller Center for Nursing Care,
    an affiliate of Montefiore Medical Center
220 West Post Road
White Plains, NY 10606

Jeanne E. Bader, PhD
Director, Center for Gerontology
University of Oregon
1607 Agate St.
Eugene, OR 97403

Lenore S. Powell, EdD, NCPsyA
Adjunct Assistant Professor of Psychology and Gerontology
College of New Rochelle
Faculty
Research Foundation of the City University of New York
161 West 12th Street
Suite 1D
New York, NY 10011

William J. Mann, MD, FACOG
Director, Division of Gynecologic Oncology
Assistant Professor, Department of Obstetrics
and Gynecology
School of Medicine
State University of New York at Stony Brook
Stony Brook, NY 11794

Lawrence R. Krakoff, MD
Professor of Medicine
Chief, Hypertension Division
Mount Sinai Medical Center
1 Gustave L. Levy Place
New York, NY 10029

Ann M. Bajart, MD
Clinical Instructor in Opthalmology
Harvard Medical School
Associate Surgeon in Ophthalmology
Massachusetts Eye and Ear Infirmary
100 Charles River Plaza
Boston, MA 02114

Frederick S. Kaplan, MD
Chief, Division of Metabolic Bone Diseases
Department of Orthopaedic Surgery
Assistant Director, the McKay Laboratory of Orthopaedic
Surgery Research
Assistant Professor of Orthopaedic Surgery
University of Pennsylvania School of Medicine
Hospital of the University of Pennsylvania
3400 Spruce Street
Philadelphia, PA 19104

Jane Porcino, PhD
Director of the Gerontology Project
Center for Continuing Education
State University of New York at Stony Brook
Stony Brook, NY 11794

Preface:
The Challenge of Women's Longevity

This special issue of *Women & Health* is devoted to the health care needs of women as they mature beyond middle age. The contributors have looked at several questions. What are the health problems that women commonly experience as they age? How are their needs being met today? And what problems are not being adequately addressed by our medical care system?

Some health problems, such as visual disorders, are faced by men and women alike. But others, such as osteoporosis and gynecological cancer are either more common or are unique to women. Health care providers need to know how these conditions can best be treated, and what preventive measures can be taken to avoid, delay, or minimize them.

The whole issue of psychosocial factors is an important one. The stereotype of old women as poor, dumb, and ugly does not make becoming an old woman a desirable fate. And we tend to see ourselves as others see us—which can be a real blow to self esteem. We need to recognize the diversity of older women to find role models to show us how to grow old successfully.

America is aging, and women more so than men. Projected death rates show an expected 9.2 year difference in female to male life expectancy by the year 2050. In an overview of demographics on health and aging, Myrna Lewis describes the acute and chronic illnesses which are associated with greater female longevity. Older women as compared to men, need more extended long term care. This is due to higher rates of widowhood and to the devastating financial consequences of longevity which puts half of elderly women near or below the poverty level. Aging women report feeling ignored and demeaned by health care providers. Indeed, their health complaints are often taken less seriously than those of aging men. Lewis stresses the need for preventive health maintenance early in life to reduce the effects of certain disorders and to detect curable illnesses in time. She notes that we have a responsibility to older women "to make later life more hospitable and habitable . . ."

Health needs relate to social policy and health care is shaped by it. Eloise Rathbone-McCuan explains that adequate health planning for the elderly must take into account projected population changes. The number of white women over age 85 is expected to increase by one and one half times in the next 30 years, while the number of black women will triple. Medical needs will be especially acute for these elderly women, many of whom will require continued long term care.

Rathbone-McCuan reviews the resources and limitations of current health care coverage through medicare, medicaid, and private health insurance plans. She notes that retirement impacts on the physical and psychological health of women as well as men, and age of retirement often alters available medical benefits. Health advocacy groups, such as the Older Women's League, are working to create greater public awareness. The goal is to modify the social security system so that it provides comprehensive and affordable health benefits to all those in need.

Dulcy Miller observes that women have had a profound influence on the evolution of nursing homes: as long term residents, as providers of home health care, and as paid professional health workers. She reviews the structure and relationships within the nursing home as a therapeutic community, and considers the role of the medical director and the allocation of staff responsibilities. Nursing homes differ from hospitals. The focus of long term health services is generally on care rather than cure. Miller points out that often families are under great stress when they turn to nursing homes. They need help in making placement decisions for aging relatives and in evaluating facilities. Community support is especially necessary when families attempt to provide home health care on an extended basis.

Increased longevity thrusts upon women the role of caregiver, a role that may be with them for most of their lives. First children, then parents, then spouses need nurturing. Alternatives must be sought and respite care is one such idea. Respite care is an attempt to offer temporary relief to people who have undertaken the tremendous task of providing extended home health care for a loved one. Such caregiving is physically and emotionally exhausting, and generally unappreciated by family, friends, and taxpayers. Jeanne Bader explains that respite care can take many forms, including short term sitters so that the caregiver can get away for a day; home visiting services provided by trained personnel; day care centers; and temporary institutionalization of the patient when the caregiver needs relief. As Bader points out, it is often cost effective to invest in respite care for the caregiver, so they can continue to serve the primary patient. Practical and policy issues along with the advantages and disadvantages of respite care are also considered in this paper.

One of the tragedies associated with increased longevity is the growing number of people who are struck down by Alzheimer's disease. Now the fourth leading cause of death among the elderly, this illness afflicts the patient, the family, and especially the primary caregiver. Lenore Powell reviews the etiology, symptoms, and progressive stages of Alzheimer's disease, including the continuously changing needs of those affected. Emphasis is placed on the problems faced by the caregivers, and their need for personal and community support.

Malignancies of the female reproductive tract are a significant threat to aging women, as well as to younger ones. William Mann reviews the incidence and treatment programs currently being used for cancer of the breast, cervix, endometrium, ovary, and vulva. A number of general and innovative therapies are noted, including parenteral nutrition and reconstructive surgery. Mann also assesses future trends in cancer management and suggests that patient education remains a very important aspect of prevention and treatment.

High blood pressure is the most common cardiovascular disorder. Lawrence Krakoff reviews sex differences in hypertensive disease noting that women tolerate hypertension better than men, and have fewer strokes and far fewer heart attacks as a result of it. Krakoff discusses the possible causes of hypertension; he observes that it tends to run in families, suggesting a strong genetic component. However, the vast majority of people suffering from high blood pressure have "essential hypertension," the cause of which remains unknown. One point of particular relevance to women is the fact that women taking oral contraceptives generally experience a small increase in arterial blood pressure; the long term effects of this remain to be established. Kaplan concludes that antihypertensive drug treatment is beneficial for both men and women who suffer from severe hypertension; however, non-drug approaches such as weight reduction, dietary change, and exercise may be equally effective in the treatment of mild hypertension.

Loss of visual capacity is a frightening prospect. Ann Bajart reviews the causes, symptomatology, preferred treatment, and overall prognosis for the four most common visual disorders: cataracts, glaucoma, macular degeneration, and dry eye syndrome. Women are subject to dry eyes and cataracts, she notes, simply because they survive to the advanced ages when these conditions naturally occur. Treatment for dry eyes consists of keeping the eyes well lubricated through artificial tears and humidification of the home. Other degenerative processes of the visual system typically occur after the 8th decade of life. Macular degeneration and glaucoma produce slow progressive changes with cumulative loss of vision. Bajart emphasizes the importance of regular eye examinations, every three years from age forty to sixty and then every one to two years thereafter. Early detection permits prompt diagnosis and aims at prevention of the progression of eye problems. Bajart also notes that there is now evidence that intense ultraviolet light increases the likelihood of cataract formation and retinal degeneration and suggests that it would be prudent to avoid intense sunlight and use ultraviolet filtering glasses as prophylactic measures.

Post menopausal women are at high risk for osteoporosis, a condition of decreased bone mass and a leading cause of fractures in the elderly. In his review, Frederick S. Kaplan notes that half the females over the age of 50 have detectable evidence to osteoporosis. There are dramatic sex differences in this condition: annual bone loss in older women is two to five times greater than in men. Sedentary women with a lifelong calcium deficiency are most susceptable. Kaplan warns that despite popular belief to the contrary, our need for calcium increases with age, yet consumption and absorption of calcium are often inadequate. The symptomatology, diagnosis, and treatment of osteoporosis are discussed along with endocrine related disorders. Risk can be reduced by insuring adequate dietary intake, and by engaging in regular weight-bearing exercise. Aging women need to be made more aware of these preventive measures.

What special psychological problems threaten the well being of aging women? Jane Porcino begins her discussion of this question by noting the double standard of aging. For instance, females are judged more harshly than males for loss of attractiveness and this can lead to social rejection and loss of self esteem. Two out of three women over 65 are unmarried, and for them, loneliness is a major challenge. Death of a mate means loss of an intimate companion, lover, provider, and practical helpmate. Porcino notes that sexual needs remain strong as women age, and often their greatest sexual problem is lack of an available partner. The loneliness of singlehood and the stresses of illness and poverty can lead some women to alcoholism and drug dependency. These addictions may be overlooked or misdiagnosed by professionals. A major source of psychological strength that helps women cope with the stresses of aging is their ability to form intimate bonds and to utilize support networks. Contributors to this special issue note that women live a long time but do not necessarily manage aging as well as they might. The editors believe that all health professionals are responsible for the fate of older women and that the special needs of women as they age can best be met by an informed population of physicians, nurses, psychologists, social workers, geriatric specialists, health educators, and public health officials. This volume moves to address the challenge of women's longevity.

Rita Jackaway Freedman, PhD
Sharon Golub, PhD

Health Needs
of Women
as They Age

Older Women and Health:
An Overview

Myrna Lewis, ACSW

ABSTRACT. Older women's health issues are unique. There are more older women than ever before. They are living increasingly longer than men, yet they report more acute and chronic illness and disability than men. They are disproportionally represented in nursing homes, since many women are alone: twenty-five percent aged 70 or over have no living children and over 60 percent of older women are widowed, divorced, or single. Older women have fewer personal financial resources for health care than men. Health care reimbursement does not meet their needs for financial coverage of chronic outpatient and nursing home care. They face age and sex discrimination on the part of many health care providers and are subject to a growing tendency to be seen as "burdens" and "problems" in the American health care system.

An American woman over 60 years of age today was born in the early 1920s or before, when medicine was virtually helpless against the infectious diseases and epidemics that claimed so many lives. The 1918-1919 flu epidemic, for example, killed an estimated half million Americans out of a population of only 100 million people (20 million persons died worldwide) before it ran its deadly course. Maternal mortality, infant mortality, and deaths from infections in general were high. In 1915-19, 730 women died per every 100,000 live births (U.S. Department Health and Human Services, 1979), compared to 8.9 per 100,000 in 1982. The mothers and grandmothers of today's older women probably knew about and may have practiced the use of typical 19th Century "cures" such as "bleeding" (opening veins and removing large quantities of blood), "cupping" (putting suction cups on the skin to "draw out" infection), violent purging of the stomach and bowels, raising blisters through use of skin-irritating ointments, immersing the body in ice cold or

Part of this article represents the author's contribution to a larger committee paper on Health and Older Women in New York State, written for the New York Statewide Conference on Older Women, held October 24-25, 1983 at Fordham University, New York City.

1

scalding hot water—all desperate and frustratingly ineffective attempts to fight disease and premature death (Thomas, 1983).

By early 1930, the causes of many infectious diseases were already well understood. The discovery of the germ theory of disease in the late 19th Century and the introduction of public hygiene measures as a result of this, brought the first impressive drops in death and disease rates, even before 1920. However, although prevention of illness improved, cure remained elusive once a disease was contracted. Bedrest, nursing care, personal hygiene, and other public health measures, combined with drugs like aspirin, morphine, cathartics, bromides, and digitalis, were the slim defenses in the battle against disease. Syphilis, tuberculosis, typhoid, rheumatic fever, erysipelas, poliomyelitis and lobar pneumonia were prominent. By mid-1930 some treatments became available for diabetes, the early stage of syphilis, and some forms of lobar pneumonia, as well as for pernicious anemia, pellegra, and diptheria. But nothing could be done for dreaded killers like tuberculosis (affecting women more than men), tertiary syphilis and, for children, rheumatic heart disease, to name a few.

The introduction of sulfa in the 1937 followed in the 1940s and 1950s by penicillin, streptomycin, chloromycetin and an array of other antibiotics marked a revolution in modern medicine. At last a treatment had been found capable of curing many infectious diseases, augmented by increasingly effective public health programs. A great many more women and their infants began to survive the process of childbirth. The population as a whole began increasingly to die from the "diseases of old age"—cancer and heart disease—rather than from infections contracted earlier in life. Medicine moved from an art which emphasized human contact, the laying on of hands and the often futile, although still comforting presence of the physician witnessing the natural progression of a disease, to a science based on technologies like laboratory testing, much faster paced medical consultations—often with teams of doctors—and quick and dramatic cures through drugs and surgery.

AMERICA IS AGING

In the 20th Century, death rates for both sexes dropped steadily until about 1940. Then White female death rates continued to decline, while White and Black male and Black female death rates rose until the 1960s. The latter rates finally began to decline again after the mid-1960s, with the new decline especially evident in heart and cerebro-vascular disease. (See Chart #1.) Explanations for the recent declines are still under question. Various interpretations crediting better control of smoking, diet, and exercise have been postulated, although not yet fully proven. Better management of hypertension and of heart disease in general as well as improved access to health care following the introduction of Medicare in 1965 are additional and perhaps even stronger factors. The consequences of falling death rates is of course a growing population of older persons. Simply put, more people live to old age. Although the maximum age attainable, about 110 years, has remained the same for two centuries, what has changed is the chance an individual has of reaching old age. In the United States the percentage of those age 65 and older rose from 4% of the population in 1900 to over 12% today with projections of 20% by the year 2020.

WOMEN ARE LIVING LONGER THAN MEN

Evidence exists that females lived an average of 2-4 years longer than males throughout much of the 19th Century in America (Armstrong, 1983). The first statistical tables, recorded in 1900, show

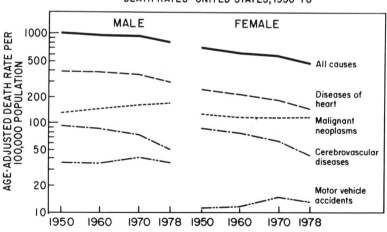

DEATH RATES: UNITED STATES, 1950-78

Source: *National Center for Health Statistics, Division of Vital Statistics*

CHART #1.

life expectancy at birth for females to be 2 years longer than for males, although at age 65 there were slightly more men (1.6 million) than women (1.5 million)—evidence of high maternal mortality in the earlier generations (U.S. Department of Health and Human Services, 1980a). In 1930 female life expectancy was 3.1 years longer than males' and in 1950, it had increased to 6.1 years. (See Chart #2.)

By 1981 the average national life expectancy for a baby girl was 77.9 years and a baby boy 70.3 years. Thus, females will live an average of 7-1/2 years longer than males. (Females have an advantage in life expectancy over males throughout the life cycle, but especially from ages 15-34, when men die at twice the rate of women. A higher rate of auto and other accidents among males and a higher use of guns and alcohol contribute to this.) Women who were already 65 years old in 1979 can expect to live an average of 18 more years; a man of 65, 14 more years. (Life expectancy for those who have already reached 65 is longer than life expectancy at birth in any given year because of the impact of infant and child mortality.) In 1982 there were 16.6 million women 65 years and older compared to only 10.7 million older men—a difference of 5.9 million additional women.

The U.S. Census Bureau projects that the difference in life expectancy between men and women may continue to increase until the year 2050 when rates will level off. At this point, life expectancy for women will be 81 years and males 71.8 years, a 9.2 year difference. (See Chart #3.) There will be 33.4 million women 65 years and older and 22.1 million older men, a difference of 11.3 million additional women. This assumes that immigration, emigration, birth, and mortality rates remain relatively predictable.

The proportion of very old women to very old men has increased faster than any other age group. Census Bureau figures and projections indicate the following:

In 1900—96.3 men per 100 women age 75+
In 1979—45 men per 100 women age 85+
By 2000—39.4 men per 100 women age 85+
By 2050—38.8 men per 100 women age 85+

This has sobering consequences in terms of the number of frail elderly women the United States can expect to have in the future, assuming current levels of disability continuing in the 85 year and older group.

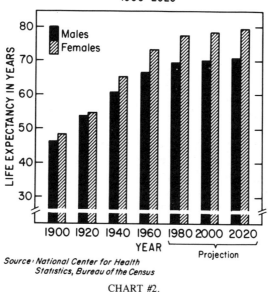

LIFE EXPECTANCY AT BIRTH-MEN AND WOMEN
1900-2020

Source: National Center for Health
Statistics, Bureau of the Census

CHART #2.

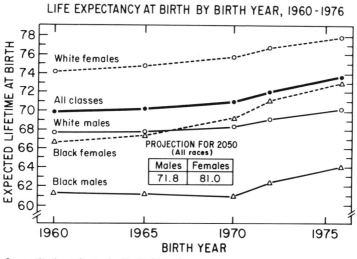

LIFE EXPECTANCY AT BIRTH BY BIRTH YEAR, 1960-1976

PROJECTION FOR 2050
(All races)

Males	Females
71.8	81.0

Source: National Center for Health Statistics,
Bureau of the Census

CHART #3.

THE REASONS FOR GREATER FEMALE LONGEVITY

If either professional experts on aging or the general public is asked why women live longer than men, a lively debate ensues between those who credit sex linked differences (women are built stronger) and those who focus on environmental stress and exposure (men are exposed to more danger). A more careful look at all the possibilities reveals a likely interplay and interaction among all of the following factors (Waldron, 1982; Verbrugge, 1983):

1. Sex-linked physical differences—one possibility is that females at all ages may have better immune resistance. Natural female hormones may also offer certain protection for women, but seemingly not for men.
2. Different exposure to environmental hazards—men's jobs may traditionally have brought them into more contact with hazards like carcinogens. It is estimated that 4 million workers, mostly men, have been or are currently exposed to asbestos and roughly 1/10 of male lung cancer deaths are related to asbestos exposure. (It has been pointed out however, that the hazards in the home environment have not been as systematically studied.)
3. Different health habits—men traditionally have smoked and used alcohol much more heavily than women. Smoking is now increasing proportionally in younger women. From 1976-1980 the proportion of smokers of both sexes has steadily declined, but the decline has been proportionally greater for males than for females. Teenage girls are beginning to start smoking in greater proportion than teenage boys. (U.S. Department of Health and Human Services, 1980b.)
4. Different personality styles—perhaps more males than females have up to this point developed what has been called "Type A Personalities"—hard-driving, competitive, and stress prone—with greater risk of ischemic (coronary) heart disease.
5. Differences in reactions to illness and disability, including knowledge about illness, behavior toward illness, and access to health care.

Evidence is growing that perhaps as much as two-thirds or more of the difference in life expectancy is related to environmental exposure, health habits, and social-cultural behavior rather than sex-linked physical differences. The overwhelming factors appear to be smoking and alcohol. A study of 4400 people, reported in *The New York Times* on 8/10/83, adds to the evidence that smoking and death by violence (accidents, homicides, and suicides) account for a large part of the male-female longevity difference. But the greater durability of the female body remains a piece of the answer. Even the vast majority of the animal world has a longer female life expectancy (Hamilton, 1948).

THE HEALTH CONSEQUENCES OF FEMALE LONGEVITY

The illness and disability patterns of women in the U.S. follow logically from their greater longevity. Since women die later in life than men, they accumulate more chronic diseases and disabilities before death. Let us look at some of the characteristic differences between the sexes.

Older women report both more acute and chronic illness and disability than older men, but die at a lesser rate. Another way of saying this is that when older men report that they are ill, they are more likely to die than women are. Some of this may be the result of women's greater freedom to report their illnesses; but the general consensus holds that women genuinely do have a greater incidence and prevalence of illness. In 1984 the National Center on Health Statistics is conducting a new health interview survey aimed at older people to update the data in this area. (See Table 1 for the most frequent chronic conditions and impairments in older women.)

Older men spend more days in hospitals per person than women (Kovar, 1984). Older women are much more likely to spend time in a nursing home or to need home care services. And older women typically have more multiple health problems, requiring coordination of care among various caregivers (the accumulation factor).

There are a number of interesting differences between older men and women in certain specific disorders, for example: women have higher rates of hypertension, but men die more frequently from it. (Some speculate that women's higher rate of doctors visits result in earlier detection and treatment.) Death rates from ischemic (coronary) heart disease are half as high for women as for men. Evidence points in a number of directions—especially heavier smoking and more Type A personalities among men. Men's lung

Table 1 Prevalence rates per 1000 population of selected chronic conditions and impairments in order of frequency for non-institutionalized women 65 years and older: United States in 1978.

Chronic Condition and Impairment		Rate per 1000 Population
Arthritis (not elsewhere classified)		522.1
Hypertensive disease (not elsewhere classified)		302.1
Hearing impairment		259.1
Visual impairment		231.0
Heart condition		190.4
Hypertensive heart disease	45.0	
Coronary heart disease	78.8	
Chronic Sinusitis		134.0
Varicose veins		97.4
Diabetes		93.9
Orthopedic impairment - back or spine		84.6
Frequent constipation		74.9
All disease of urinary system		70.8
Orthopedic impairment - Lower extremity and hip		70.6
Corns and callosities		69.0
Diseases of nail		61.7
Chronic bronchitis		55.2
Hernia of abdominal cavity		49.8
Functional and symptomatic upper gastrointestinal disorder		49.2
All thyroid conditions		41.8
Diverticula of intestine		40.7
All anemia conditions		35.1
Cerebrovascular disease		34.6
Gall bladder condition		29.5
Intestional condition		20.4
Emphysema		20.2
Chronic enteritis and ulcerative colitis		18.2
Migraine		18.1

Source: Adapted from unpublished data from the 1978 National Health Interview Survey. National Center for Health Statistics.

cancer incidence and mortality rates, largely connected to smoking and/or environmental exposure, especially asbestos, far exceed those of women, but women's rates have been increasing since the 1960s—reflecting an increase in female smoking beginning in the 1930s. Lung cancer is moving ahead of breast cancer as the leading cause of cancer death in women. Other than cancers related to smoking, the difference in rate of deaths from cancer is small between the sexes, although the type of cancer varies. Men lead in orthopedic problems until age 65 and then women lead, largely due to osteoporosis (bone-thinning). Women have for years had a higher incidence of and mortality from diabetes than men, but mortality rates now are only slightly higher than men, probably due to better medical management (U.S. Department of Health and Human Services, 1982).

It is hypothesized that health habits other than the obvious ones of smoking and excess alcohol use may play a role, although a much lesser one in female longevity. Some speculate that women may be more aware of symptoms at an earlier stage and may be more likely to visit a doctor, restrict activity, or take time off for a given illness. On the other hand, evidence is beginning to accumulate that women delay as long as men in potentially life-threatening situations, such as the discovery of cancer symptoms. Women also may have more experience with and an inclination toward self care since most have been the family nurses, caring for other family members including older persons. Still others believe women may be more acculturated to cooperate rather than to compete, resulting in less stress-prone behavior and health breakdown.

LONG TERM CARE FOR OLDER WOMEN

Older women make much greater use than older men of long-term care institutions—primarily nursing homes—as well as home and community-based long-term care. About 75% of nursing home residents are females. The reasons for this are relatively straight forward:

1. Women live longer—(5% of all elderly over 65 are in institutions, but of those over 85, 22% are institutionalized).
2. Women outlive spouses while men are usually taken care of by their wives.
3. Accumulating disabilities may finally overwhelm women if they are alone or those caring for them can no longer handle the deterioration of ability to function.
4. Organic brain conditions propel many into nursing homes (over 50% of residents have serious organic brain syndromes—OBS) and more women have OBS than men because of their longevity and greater numbers.
5. About 50% of U.S. women in nursing homes are childless or have outlived their children. Twenty-five percent of all women

around 70, in and out of institutions, have no living children.
This is the low-fertility generation of the Great Depression.
6. Female caregivers in their 40s and 50s or older are increasingly in the work force and unable to care for sick relatives requiring nursing and/or custodial care. The least expensive
form of care for the old has typically been an available middle-
generation female. Now this resource is disappearing into the
outside work force.
7. It is now entirely possible for 5 or even 6 generations to be
alive in one family. A 40 year old woman may have a 60 year
old mother and father and an 80 year old grandmother, as well
as a great-grandmother and perhaps her mate's relatives to
care for. This in addition to her children in their 20s and possi-
bly, very young grandchildren. Thus, even if women were not
moving into the paid work force, the middle generation of
women (since women usually do the physical caretaking, although men may share the financial responsibilities), clearly
cannot always sustain the growing number of older relatives
likely to need care and support.

THE FINANCIAL CONSEQUENCES
OF FEMALE LONGEVITY

The greater longevity of women has health care financing consequences both for women's personal lives and for social and health
policy at all levels. The central fact is that older women have fewer
personal financial resources for health care than older men and these
resources must be spread out over a longer life time. Medicare, the
program begun in 1965 for the purpose of financing health care for
the old, pays about 40% of average health care costs. The rest of the
costs must come from private insurance or from older people themselves. Since the total median income for older women in 1983 was
only $108.00 per week or $5,599.00 a year, compared to $9,766.00
for older men, there is little available for out-of-pocket medical expenses (Patterson, 1984).

The median annual income for older women is just $800.00 over
the U.S. official poverty level; therefore, the majority of women are
either already in poverty or perilously close to it. Forty-three percent of all older females, mostly widows, live alone or with non-

relatives, and of this group nearly 30% are in official poverty (Grossman, 1984). This includes many of the very old and frail. There is almost no comparable category of males since their incomes are much higher and most live with mates or in families. Nearly half of Black older women, one quarter of Hispanic and over 15 percent of White older women live below the official poverty level. As can be seen, minority older women have a proportionally higher chance of poverty and are the poorest of the poor; but the vast majority of the poor elderly are older White women. A unique feature of old age is that women who were poor all their lives are joined by the "newly poor"—the middle class and even upper class women who may sink to the poverty level, depending upon whether they outlive their resources or, more likely, experience catastrophic or chronic illnesses requiring expensive care. Few, for example, can afford the costs of long-term care, in or out of institutions. Nursing home costs alone can amount to three to five thousand dollars per month.

Medicare was designed through its reimbursement structure to encourage acute, inpatient care rather than the chronic outpatient and long-term care more typically needed by women. To illustrate, Medicare does not cover prescription drugs, eyeglasses, hearing aids, dental services, routine physical examinations and foot care, long-term home care or, most significantly, nursing home care. In short, the illness and disability patterns of older women are not adequately reflected in the nation's major health reimbursement plan for the old.

When costs for health care rise beyond capacity to pay, women must first spend their overall resources down to the poverty level—in New York State a woman is allowed to keep $2600.00 in assets (with a number of exceptions and exemptions possible). Many other states allow even less. When the required poverty level has been reached, women can then apply for Medicaid, the state-federal "welfare" program for financing health care for the poor. Ideally, the older woman must time her application for Medicaid to match her last illness before death. If not, her recovery means that she has almost no assets, other than any pensions she collects, to live out the rest of her life.

The greater longevity of women means that a significant number of married couples already "spend down" to the Medicaid level to obtain financing for the husband's dying days. This can mean that the widow is then left in poverty for 15 or more years unless she is one of the fortunate few with a substantial pension.

OLDER WOMEN'S EXPERIENCES
WITH THE HEALTH CARE SYSTEM

Many older woman regard physicians with a certain reverence and awe. The growing technology of science-based medicine, especially the development of antibiotics and improved diagnostic and surgical procedures began occurring in their early lives and understandably, must have been impressive. At the same time, women lost an important role as medical practitioners in their own families as well as in the larger world. Until the early part of the 20th Century female lay healers and midwives were prominent in the practice of medicine (in 1910, 50% of babies had been delivered by midwives). Women physicians were able to find training opportunities in some medical schools and hospitals. But with the "professionalization" of medicine after about 1910, (with the Flexner Report demanding higher standards), only the largest and most rigorous medical schools survived and these for the most part excluded women, Blacks, and the majority of the lower class unable to afford the newly required extensive education. Medicine became White, male, and middle-class. State licensing laws swiftly excluded midwives from obstetrical practice, and except for the very important role of nursing, today's older women were relegated to the role of the consumers of health care.

Whether in relatively good health or in need of home care or institutionalized care, older women's experience as consumers in the health care system is marked too frequently by reports by women themselves of neglect and disrespect. Their chronic diseases are often ignored or undertreated, as medicine occupies iteself with more acute conditions. Physicians tend to belittle their complaints and symptoms by attributing them to "post menopausal syndrome," old age, hypochondriasis or other neurotic behaviors, "senility," or by over-prescribing tranquilizers and other medications in the belief that many physical complaints of older women are psychosomatic in origin. For example, according to the 1978 President's Commission on Mental Health, 67% of prescriptions for psychotropic drugs, like valium and librium, were for women.

By definition, chronic conditions, especially when they are newly developing, are more subtle than acute ailments. Especially with older women, physicians who dismiss their symptoms as "unspecific" miss the challenge of diagnosing and treating less-than-obvious presenting conditions. There is a saying among women that "if an older women goes to the doctor she gets a valium, an older man gets a work-up.'' The following are some typical responses gathered by New York University Medical Center when the Division of Gerontology distributed 10,000 questionnaires nationally to older women and received 1200 replies to the request to ''share any experience you have had with the health care system'': ''. . . anything the matter with you 'is to be expected at your age' ''; ''I do not feel the health care system accords older persons appropriate respect''; ''I have been treated as a non-person, with boundless time to wait . . .''

Discrimination jeopardizes the medical care of older lesbian and minority-group women. Mates of older gay women are seldom acknowledged as significant relationships and may be excluded from supportive roles in the care of the sick person. Access to all areas of health care is difficult for minority older women, especially those who are poor and unable to speak English. Rural older women also suffer from lack of services, especially transportation services to medical facilities. Inner city women may be trapped in their homes by fear of crime, lack of money or transportation, or lack of a traveling companion if they are frail.

Older women who are in institutions or are receiving home care encounter other problems. Those providing their basic care, the majority of whom are female, are often underpaid and undertrained, and seldom have the opportunity to resolve their own personal feelings about working with the sick elderly. Health care workers of all kinds struggle with anxieties about dependency, suffering, and death as they care for the old. In addition, they must provide care in the context of a society filled with negative attitudes toward women as they age. The ugly witch, the complaining ''kvetch,'' the nagging mother-in-law, and the ''senile old lady'' are some of the common images of older women, tempered by stereotypes that err on the other side—the unbelievably benevolent ''rocking chair grandma'' who bakes cookies on cue and the docile, helpless older woman who makes no demands, is able to live uncomplainingly on a pittance, and is a perfect target for muggers and rip-off artists. There is little recognition of the value of older women's lifetime contributions to society. Their work is not considered part of the gross national product. Their accumulated wisdom, survival skills, range of personality, and creativity are seldom acknowledged. It is not surprising therefore, that health care workers often reflect the larger cultural disregard and even disdain for older women.

EDUCATION AND RESEARCH
ON OLDER WOMEN'S HEALTH

The major textbooks on geriatric medicine pay scant attention to the medical implications of females living longer than males. Nor do they attach much import to the question of whether women age differently than men, even at the same ages. The "unisex" quality of current geriatric medical literature represents a lag in recognizing the clinical implications of the differences between males and females. Medical and epidemiological research reflect the same lag. Many studies have excluded women altogether. One of the most important, the Baltimore Longitudinal Study of Aging, has examined men for over 20 years, but did not include women until 1978. The National Institute of Mental Health's landmark work on healthy aging, published in 1963, involved only men (Birren, Butler, Greenhouse, Sokoloff, & Yarrow, 1963). Certain processes common to all women as they age remain mysterious; for example there is no agreement yet on the basic physiology of the menopausal hot flash. On a more urgent level, the breast cancer death rates in the United States have not improved in twenty years (Kovar, 1984).

Certain health conditions can be singled out as immediate targets for major new or expanded research efforts because of their impact on so many older women and because of current controversy around treatment—Alzheimer's Disease, breast cancer, uterine cancer, hypertension, stroke, osteoporosis (brittle bones), diabetes, arthritis, and urinary incontinence are some of the most apparent. Further research around the use of estrogens, hysterectomies, and mastectomies is indicated. As already mentioned, the menopause and post-menopausal period requires greater understanding. Occupational health hazards for women, both in the home and in the outside work place, warrant further examination. Better understanding and prevention of hypothermia (dangerously low body temperature) and heat stroke are important, especially for the frail elderly.

The Importance of Health Maintenance for Older Women

The maintenance of "wellness" and self care needs emphasis among mid-life and older women. Simple measures like sleeping 7-8 hours a night, controlling weight (not more than 10% over standard desirable weight for females), exercising, no more than moderate use of alcohol, and no smoking can produce significantly better health and lower mortality, according to a study by the California State Health Department (U.S. Department of Health and Human Services, 1982). Campaign efforts against smoking must begin in the teenage years when most women start smoking. The midlife period is critical for developing preventive habits against such disorders as osteoporosis and hypertension, and for early detection of diseases like breast and uterine cancer. Informal and formal education of women in these areas will not only produce better health, but also could spare enormous health costs. It is likely that self care, prevention, and early detection of disease will represent a major next advance in American health—no longer simply a question of individual choice, but a critical factor in reducing the enormous personal and public health care costs which currently face us.

CONCLUSION

Although older women's health is not yet seen as a viable, separate field of study, the demographics of population aging and the growing differences in life expectancy between men and women make this a natural direction for research, education, clinical practice and health policy. We are witnessing an exciting revolution in the survival of increasing numbers of people into old age, and older women are leading the way by being the first large group of those survivors. We still have much to learn from them about the adaptations they are learning to make to the old age that many of us who are younger will also eventually face. We also have a responsibility to work together with older women to make later life more hospitable and habitable—by confronting poverty, an absurdly expensive health care system that does not adequately meet older women's most common health needs, and a cultural prejudice which still fails to recognize the work and contributions of older women.

REFERENCES

Armstrong, R. (1983). Personal communication. Actuarial advisor, Life Expectancy Division, National Center of Health Statistics.

Birren, J. E., Butler, R. N., Greenhouse, S. W., Sokoloff, L., & Yarrow, M. R. (1963. Reprinted 1971, 1974). *Human aging: A biological and behavioral study.* U.S. Public Health Service Publication No. 986, Washington, D.C.: U.S. Government Printing Office.

Grossman, K. (1984). Personal communication. Statistician, Poverty Statistics, Population Division, Bureau of the Census.

Hamilton, J. B. (1948). Role of testicular secretions as indicated by the effects of castration in man and by studies of pathological conditions and the short lifespan associated with maleness. In G. Pincus (Ed.) *Recent progress in hormone research* (pp. 257-322). New York: Academic Press.

Kovar, M. G. (1984). Personal communication. Senior Statistics, National Center of Health Statistics. See also National Center of Health Statistics, Breast cancer death rates for women ages 35-44, 1960-1980. Division of Vital Statistics.

Patterson, G. (1984). Personal communication. Income Section, U.S. Bureau of Census.

Thomas, L. (1983). *The youngest science: Notes of a medicine watcher.* New York: Viking Press.

U.S. Department of Health and Human Services (1979). Mortality statistics, 1915-19, in *Vital Statistics,* Vol. II. National Center on Health Statistics.

U.S. Department of Health and Human Services (1980a). *Life Tables,* Vol. II, Section 5, Table 5-5, Vital Statistics of the United States. Washington, D.C.: U.S. Government Printing Office.

U.S. Department of Health and Human Services (1980b). *Surgeon General's report on the health consequences of smoking for women.* Public Health Service: Office on Smoking and Health.

U.S. Department of Health and Human Services (1982). Basic data from Wave II of the national survey of personal health practices and consequences: U.S. 1980. National Center of Health Statistics, Working papers.

U.S. Department of Health and Human Services (1982). Unpublished data on the 15 leading causes of death, 65 years of age and older in 1979. National Center of Health Statistics.

Verbrugge, L. M. (1983). Women and men: Mortality and health of older people. In M. W. Riley, B. B. Hess, & K. Bond (Eds.) *Aging in society* (pp. 139-174). Hillsdale, New Jersey: Lawrence Erlbaum Associates.

Waldron, I. (1982). An analysis of causes of sex differences in mortality and morbidity. In W. R. Gove & G. R. Carpenter (Eds.) *The fundamental connections between nature and nurture* (pp. 69-116). Lexington, Mass.: Lexington Books.

Health Needs and Social Policy

Eloise Rathbone-McCuan, PhD

ABSTRACT. This article describes demographic and economic factors that impinge on the health care of elderly women. Policies that control access to and utilization of health and long term care services are discussed. Some of the shortcomings of past policies are noted and current social reform efforts aimed at greater policy equity for elder women are reviewed.

DEMOGRAPHICS OF THE AGING FEMALE POPULATION

Much of the current concern over health issues of older women is related to those living to very advanced old age, usually defined as 75 years and older. In 1982, the life expectancy of females was 78.2 years and was almost 8 years longer than the life expectancy of men. Table 1 indicates the projected growth rates of numbers of women between 1990 and 2020. By 2010, in less than 30 years, the number of white females 85 years and over is expected to increase about 1-1/2 times while the number of black females will triple. The social policies that are operating now have most direct impact on the women who have reached the age of benefit entitlement. However, future cohorts of women tend to be ignored because American social policy is reactive rather than proactive.

Two areas of social policy having implications for older women are housing/living arrangements and income maintenance. Table 2 shows the distribution of living arrangements of older women in America. Widowhood leads to the high proportion of women living alone and that trend rises dramatically with increasing age.

Housing is the single largest budget item for older women (Porcino, 1983). With increasing pressure on older women to let go of their family home (Howell, 1982) and serious rent inflation combined with a loss of rent subsidy (Storey, 1983), housing is often a crisis of great proportion. Yet Federal government policy does not

Table 1

Projected Trends in Size of Older Female Population 1990-2020

(in millions and percentage)

Females	1990	2000	2010	2020
55-64	108 (8.6%)	12.1 (9.0%)	17.1 (12.1%)	19.3 (12.9%)
65-74	10.1 (8.1%)	9.8 (7.3%)	11.0 (7.8%)	15.6 (10.4%)
75+	7.8 (6.2%)	9.3 (7.0%)	9.8 (6.9%)	11.0 (7.3%)

Source: U.S. Bureau of the Census, "Projections of the Population of
           the United States: 1977 to 2050," Current Population
           Reports, Series P-25, No. 704.

Table 2

Living Arrangements of Older Women in

United States in 1979[1]

	Living With Spouse	Living Alone	Living With Relatives Other	Living With NonRelative
Females				
65 - 74	47%	35%	15%	2%
75 & Older	21%	50%	27%	2%

[1]
Excludes females 65 and older living in institutions.

Source: U.S. Bureau of the Census, "Marital Status and Living
           Arrangements: March 1981, February 1980 Current Population
           Reports, Series D-20. 349.

treat housing as an entitlement. The projection of special government support for housing to be available by 1985 is more than four
million units. Based on the projected need, the supply may be able to
meet the needs of 25 percent of the elderly who qualify for these
units. At this time the U.S. Department of Housing and Urban De-

velopment (HUD) and the Farmers Home Administration (FHA) show only a minimal interest in this dramatic housing shortfall. Over the past 30 years there has been improvement in the annual cash income of the elderly. Nevertheless, income inadequacy remains great and deficiencies are more serious for older women than older men. Table 3 shows the increasing incidence of poverty among women associated with progressing age. The issue of poverty for older women takes on a more critical position when one includes statistics on the poverty level of minority older women. There are conditions of triple jeopardy facing older Hispanics. These are related to the interactive conditions of poverty, language barriers, and minority group status (Lacayo, 1982). The heightened risk also extends to black elders; and elderly females in both minority groups experience these situations more than their shorter living male counterparts (Eaglin, 1982). Thus the feminization of poverty is vividly felt by minority older women and cannot be ignored as a major health risk.

The percentage of women who are employed in the paid labor force has steadily increased since World War II (King & Marvel, 1982). In 1983, 4.8 million women aged 55 to 64 were in the labor force compared to 7.2 million men. Table 4 shows the percentage increase of women in the labor force. As of 1983, there were

Table 3

Incidence of Poverty among Women Age

55 and Older, by Race, 1981

Percentage of Older Women with
Income Below Poverty Line

	Age 55-64	Age 65 and Older
Females	12.1	18.6
White Females	9.9	16.2
Black Females	33.7	43.5
Hispanic Females	21.2	27.4

Source: U.S. Bureau of the Census, "Money Income and Poverty
Status of Families and Persons in the United States:
1981," Current Population Reports, Series, P-60,
No. 134.

Table 4

Percentage Trends of Older Women In

Labor Force 1950 - 1980

	1950	1955	1960	1965	1970	1975	1980
Females							
55 - 64	27.0	32.5	37.2	41.1	43.0	41.0	41.5
65+	9.7	10.6	10.8	10.0	9.7	8.3	8.1

Source: U.S. Department of Labor, "Employment and Training Report of the President" (Washington, D.C.: GPO, 1982)

notable differences in the numbers of women employed in both age groups. There were 3,264,000 women age 55 to 64 employed full time and only 453,000 employed in the older cohort. Employment, however, does not assure economic stability. Work history greatly influences both private and public pension structures and transfer payment problems. Solutions connected to policy formulations include both short range policies, such as greater income support for women who have completed their work careers, and long range plans involving better pension coverage and job opportunities (O'Rand & Henretta, 1982). There is agreement between economists and older women's advocates that issues of adequacy and equity of benefits to older men as compared to older women require policy reform (Rathbone-McCuan, 1982).

THE HEALTH IMPLICATIONS OF RETIREMENT

Greater numbers of working women demand greater attention to the retirement needs of women. Szinovacz (1982) reviewed the few studies that examined retirement as an aging issue among women. The interrelationship between women's health and retirement is relevant to the types of services they need. For example, it is rarely noted that older women do leave employment because of disabilities; this creates a need for benefits before the usual retirement age.

It is increasingly difficult to justify social insurance programs for disability toward which women pay taxes, but whose benefits are unavailable to them (Mudrick, 1983). Both physical and emotional disabilities contribute to withdrawal from the work role. Far more research is needed to understand how symptoms such as pain, fatigue, disorientation, and drug misuse are linked to the working environment of women. Simple, diagnostic labeling does not adequately explain complex patterns of inability to continue work. A preventive strategy for future benefit structures for women in post-retirement years includes preparation for retirement. Older women who are close to a point of eligibility for early retirement may experience pressure from their work environment to "get out early." They may also be pressured by their spouses who retire in advance of their wives and urge them to leave jobs before the point where they are able to take advantage of the full range of benefits. Many variables influence how women prepare or fail to prepare for retirement. Kroeger (1982) reported that while women do participate in retirement planning their preparation differs from that of their male co-workers. Unlike women, men use multiple sources of information about retirement and engage in preparatory activities over a one to five year period before actual retirement. Women, especially nonprofessional women, approach preparation as a last minute thing, almost immediately before they retire. Thus the research indicates a need for better efforts to target women in lower income groups so that they have a longer period to plan their post retirement incomes and to establish a clear benefit plan. Policies could also encourage a diversified sponsorship of retirement planning so that women can obtain information even if their employer does not have retirement preparation services.

The retirement issues that most concern professional and nonprofessional women differ (Price-Bonham & Johnson, 1983). Those working in professional categories, often feel economically secure but worry extensively about post retirement roles and activities, while nonprofessional women are preoccupied with income security. There is a lack of adequate research on the long range effect on the health of those dissatisfied with retirement lifestyles. To the extent that retirement leads to a loss of meaningful activities and relationships and produces isolation and general disinterest, health may be impaired (Rathbone-McCuan & Hashimi, 1982).

LIMITATIONS OF CURRENT HEALTH CARE COVERAGE

Medicare, Medicaid, private insurance sources, and personal income are the major resources available to cover health care costs. There are serious limitations to some forms of coverage and this increases the risks of insufficient and inadequate care. Some groups of advocates for the elderly are confronting this problem, for example, a limited, but important reform effort is being mounted by the Older Women's League.

A. Medicare

Medicare (Title XVIII of the Social Security Act passed in 1965) is an insurance program administered by the federal government. It is available to all people eligible for Social Security, however some elderly women do not qualify for Social Security. To have maximum coverage an individual must have parts A and B because they cover different types of care. The Hospital Insurance Program, Part A, covers inpatient hospitalization, skilled nursing care, and home care if there is medical justification. Sometimes the conditions faced by the elderly woman necessitate home care, but Medicare won't cover the cost because the nature of her need doesn't fit medical justifications. Supplementary Medical Insurance Program, Part B, is voluntary and financed by federal funds and monthly contributions by those enrolled. If purchased, it covers physician services, outpatient therapy, medical equipment and home health visits. Both Parts A and B involve beneficiary payment of various deductibles and coinsurance costs (Harrington, 1983; Muse & Sawyer, 1982). Medicare has been a major source of physician directed and hospital based care for the aged (Vladeck & Forman, 1983). Of the total Medicare expenditures in 1981, almost three-quarters were spent on hospital services and one quarter on physician services. In that same year, coverage for nursing home and home healthcare was negligible (Waldo & Gibson, 1982).

B. Medicaid

Medicaid (Title XIX of the Social Security Act passed in 1965) was designed according to public welfare models. Eligibility is determined based on criteria and procedures that vary from state to state. Elderly women living in different states can expect more or less coverage, depending on limits set by her state of residence. The very poorest of elderly women depend on this funding source to a large extent. Funds cover inpatient hospital, physicians, dentists, other professional services, the range of nursing home care levels, laboratory and x-ray, home health, drugs, and mental health hospitals and clinics. Greatest expenditures occur for general hospital, skilled and intermediate nursing home care, physician services, and drug costs (Harrington, 1983). The reality of great public cost for long term care for elderly women is reflected in annual Medicaid expenditures.

C. Private Health Insurance

Little data is available about the specific role that private insurance coverage plays in the health care costs of older women. Access to and coverage under private insurance sources for aged females is most frequently associated with policies connected to the spouse. The changing employment patterns of women reflect increasing job related coverage separate from spouse-based protection. Millions of elderly women have no type of private insurance, they are not eligible and cannot afford its cost. If covered, women may realize help in paying the cost of hospital services, some physician fees, dental costs. These sources currently mean very little assistance for long term coverage. If the federal government continues to pursue competitive approaches to contain health care costs, private health insurance involvement may increase dramatically with unpredictable outcomes.

ADVOCACY ACTIVITIES

It is little wonder that elderly women fear a fate which brings them to the point where they are very frail, have outlived their family, and have lost their income reserves. Life as a Medicaid patient in a nursing home, without an informal support system of personal care, is a bleak existence and one about which older women should not remain silent.

Public pressure on issues facing older women, including both middle aged and aged women, have been largely undertaken by broader based national advocacy organizations devoted to the concerns of older people. It was not until the White House Mini Conference on Older Women, held in Des Moines, Iowa, October 1980, that the need to create a separate advocacy for older women's concerns emerged. It was formed in 1980 under the auspices of a California based coalition of older women advocates (Older Women's League, 1983). Currently there are 8000 chartered members in 30 state chapters with a Washington based legislative office and a national branch office in Oakland, California.

Since its inception, the primary concerns of OWL have included improvement of women's access to affordable health care. An important function of the Older Women's League is information sharing about the different health trends of men and women and their different health care needs. One important difference that is vital to the health of older women is their greater need for long term care. As compared to their female counterparts, older men have higher rates of fatal disease, more hospital days of care, and higher hospital fatality rates. A larger proportion of older women than men are transferred from hospitals to other facilities for continued care.

The points of the 1982 Older Women's League advocacy were clearly felt in modifications of Social Security Amendments that closed major gaps creating inequality for women. The organization documented and testified about the problem of women's medical dependency on their spouses; loss of coverage that occurred through divorce or death of the spouse; hardships created through having to pay high enrollment costs out of reach for most older women; and their inability to cover the unreimbursed aspects of their health care.

Modest gains have been made in creating equity for older women through shifts in coverage through Medicare entitlement. OWL continues to advocate for other health related concerns. For example, the tendency of much health care to be highly medicalized and lacking in reliance on ambulatory or non hospital procedures while at the same time remaining inadequality reimbursed if provided out of hospital. Another issue is the lack of education. It is important for older women to become knowledgeable consumers of health care, thus, reducing their vulnerability to fraud and the likelihood of inappropriate health consumer behaviors. Catastrophic health insurance geared to hospitalized care situations and the associated copayments that have been proposed for catastrophic health insurance is another concern (Older Women's League, 1983).

The four major issues around which the Older Women's League advocacy takes place include: the vulnerabilities of older women to all aspects of inadequacies in the long term system; the lack of public policy conceptualizations adjusted to the increased realities of older women living alone for extended periods; conditions surrounding all aspects of older women's care giving; and the conditions under which they must be cared for by others.

All of the legislative issues raised or supported by the Older

Women's League press for better coordination of acute and long term care, including pooling Medicare coverage for diversified and expanded home health care (including reimbursed costs for respite care). Issues of availability of non-institutional services and the quality of care provided in these settings overlaps with all of the long term care issues that face older women. Expansion of particular services, such as geriatric day care and day health program, are supported for national expansion and third party reimbursement because of their dual value for those needing care as well as those needing respite from care (Sommers & Shields, 1980).

These specific legislative activities are built upon a framework for health promotion and health awareness for older women that is also supported by the Gray Panthers and other groups. The long and difficult process of fostering a concern about ageism and sexism provides a unifying theme around which older women in many different organizations can unite.

It was through the efforts of these diverse groups that some corrective legislation was added into the 1983 Social Security Amendments to address problems of older women. Harrington (1983) reported that Congress did make policy changes that would continue to pay benefits for spouses who remarry, permit divorced spouses to receive benefits whether or not the insured spouse retired, provide indexing for survivor benefits by wages instead of prices, and gradually increase benefits for disabled widows and widowers aged 50 to 59 to the level payable to their counterparts 60 years and older.

CONCLUSION

Forecasting the future is very difficult. Assuming that demographic predictions of greater numbers of very old women needing expensive prolonged care and limited ability to control care costs, the current problem will become a greater crisis. One alternative might be to reconceptualize "catastrophic" coverage and have it cover the cost of care for the very oldest and most impaired who linger-in-life. For elderly women, this is a more realistic definition of a catastrophic situation. In one sense, there will be a gender split in care of men who are eligible war veterans and women and noneligible men. The proportion of elderly men needing extensive medical care through the Veteran's Administration is rapidly increasing. This may prove to be an issue of competition for Federal dollars to support long term care.

Changing the system is a popular objective for both conservative and liberal advocates. Their advocacy, once directed toward the federal government, is going to expand more toward state and local units of government. Forces attempting to better the health care of older women through prevention and intervention service expenditures should become more active at the local level. Their local targets should be private as well as public funded service sources. The quality of care provided is also an important issue. Exclusive attention to access will not address deficiences in the quality.

Efforts to change the financing and operation of the health care system through competitive approaches are being discussed. If health maintenance organizations become more available, then attempts should be made to assure that older women have equal access. Voucher system access would require that older women become educated enough to evaluate and screen their use of health services. Cost containment through employer contributions will affect greater numbers of employed older women. It is essential that all strategies be fully assessed for their impact on older women prior to implementation. Otherwise, current inadequacies may be traded for new ones even more disadvantageous to aged women.

REFERENCES

Eaglin, J. P. (1982). The nation's black elders: This is not progress. *Generations, 6*, 29-30.

Harrington, C. (1983). Social security and medicare: Policy shifts in the 1980s. In C. L. Estes & R. J. Newcomer (Eds.) *Fiscal austerity and aging*. Beverly Hills: Sage Publications.

Howell, S. (1982). Crisis for elders: House, home or shelter. *Generations, 6*, 42-43.

King, N. R., & Marvel, M. G. (1982). *Issues, policies and programs for midlife and older women*. Washington, D.C.: Center for Women Policy Studies.

Kroeger, N. (1982). Preretirement preparation: Sex differences in access, sources and use. In M. Szinovacz (Ed.), *Women's retirement*, (pp. 95-112). Beverly Hills: Sage Publication.

Lacayo, C. G. (1982). Triple jeopardy: Underserved hispanic elders. *Generations, 6*, 25-26.

Mudrick, N.R. (1983). Income support programs for disabled women. *Social Service Review, 57*, 125-136.

Muse, D. N., & Sawyer, D. (1982). The medicare and medicaid data book, 1981. Baltimore: Department of Health and Human Services, Health Care Financing Administration.

Older Women's League (1983). *A statement on longterm care* (Older Women's League, National Office testimony report). Washington, D.C.: Author.

O'Rand, A., & Henretta, J. C. (1982). Midlife work history and retirement income. In M. Szinovacz (Ed.), *Women's retirement*, (pp. 25-44). Beverly Hills: Sage Publications.

Porcino, J. (1983). *Growing older: Getting better*. Reading, Massachusetts: Addison-Wesley Publishing Company.

Price-Bonham, S., & Johnson, C. K. (1983). Attitudes toward retirement: A comparison of professional and nonprofessional married women. In M. Szinovacz (Ed.), *Women's retirement*, (pp. 123-138). Beverly Hills: Sage Publications.

Rathbone-McCuan, E. R., & Hashimi, J. (1982). *Isolated elders.* Rockville: Aspen Systems Corp.

Rathbone-McCuan, E. (1982). Older women: Endangered but surviving species. *Generations, 6,* 11-12.

Sommers, T., & Shields, L. (1980). *Older women and health care: Strategy for survival* (Gray Paper #3). Washington, D.C.: Older Women's League.

Storey, J. R. (1983). *Older American's in the Reagan era: Impacts of federal policy changes.* Washington, D.C.: Urban Institute Press.

Szinovacz, M. (1982). Research on Women's Retirement. In M. Szinovacz (Ed.), *Women's retirement,* (pp. 9-12). Beverly Hills: Sage Publications.

Valdeck, B. C., & Forman, J. P. (1983). The aging of the population and health services. *The Annals, 468,* 132-148.

Waldo, D. R., & Gibson, R. M. (1982). National health expenditures, 1981. *Health Care Financing Review, 4,* 1-35.

Women and Long Term Nursing Care

Dulcy B. Miller, MS

ABSTRACT. Women have played a significant role in long term care: formerly as volunteer caregivers and presently as volunteer and paid caretakers, as professionals working in the field and increasingly as old, old residents in nursing homes. The goal in long term care is helping people to function to their maximal level; it is based on a philosophy of care not cure. Family-patient relationships influence quality in long term facilities where nursing is the matrix of professional services. Respite care is designed to provide relief to family caretakers for time limited periods and long term home health care is a non-institutional alternative where the nursing home therapeutic regimen is brought into the patients' own home. Whatever the model, the female influence is pervasive.

Women have had a profound influence on the development of nursing homes by both their presence and their absence. In past eras when families and homes were larger, there was always room for a sick old relative and there was a housewife at home to watch out for him/her. However, with increased urbanization, families have become dispersed and increasing numbers of women have joined the work force, leaving the ill aged exposed. Of particular relevance has been the rapid entrance of middle aged women, the traditional caregivers to elderly parents, into the work force. To further exacerbate the situation, the declining birth rate has resulted in a lower ratio of potential caretakers for the oldest of the older population (Brody, Johnson, Fulcomer & Lang, 1983).

Some of the women who left home to seek employment were untrained housewives. Instead of working in domestic positions, which have lost favor in this egalitarian society, many sought employment in nursing care facilities where the preponderance of personnel are females. It is paradoxical that in former years the same women remained at home and served as caretakers to ill elderly relatives and

Requests for reprints may be addressed to the author at White Plains Center for Nursing Care, 220 West Post Road, White Plains, New York 10606.

29

now many are paid to perform the same tasks. To further compound the care problem. Brotman predicts that by the year 2,000 the ratio of women to men over 75 will be 191 to 100 (Brotman, 1977). The numbers clearly demonstrate the availability of wives to care for ill husbands in contrast to the paucity of husband survivors to care for sick spouses, making nursing home placement the only viable alternative for females. Thus, widowhood, longevity of women, the declining birth rate, absence of female caretakers, and middle aged women entering the work force have impacted on the growth of the nursing home.

In 1984, 2.6 million Americans are reported to be 85 or older. By the year 2000 it is anticipated that 5.1 million will live to age 85 or more (Long Term Care Management, 1984). What are the health care implications for anticipated 900% growth of the old old population in only 50 years? Currently 25% of those over 85 are in nursing homes as compared to only 4-5% of persons over 65. The 4-5% figure is misleading, as 20% of this younger cohort (65 and over) will spend time in a nursing home although on any given day only 4-5% will be institutionalized (Kastenbaum & Candy, 1973).

The elderly who are 85 or more have the greatest need for long term care services whether provided in the nursing home setting or in the community. Skilled nursing facility services are designed for persons who need skilled nursing care (provided directly or under the supervision of skilled nursing personnel) or other skilled rehabilitation services that on a practical level can only be provided on an inpatient basis in a skilled nursing facility (Health Care Financing Administration, 1979).

PATIENT POPULATION TO BE FOUND IN THE LONG TERM CARE FACILITY

The nursing home population consists of aged, chronically ill patients with multi-organ pathology, 80 years or older, white, predominantly female with incomes below the poverty line, and eight or fewer years of schooling (Corman, 1976). Only 10% have a living spouse and over half have no close relatives. According to Branch, living alone is the major determinant for nursing home admission among the chronically ill elderly (Branch & Jette, 1982). Two distinct patterns of nursing home length of stay have been identified. For 91% the mean stay is 2-1/2 years. For the 10% who improve or die in a brief period, the mean stay is 1 year 8 months (Keeler, Kane, & Soloman, 1981).

While many nursing home admissions result from medical illnesses such as strokes, heart disease, hip fractures, etc., in 70-80% of the cases the major management problem relates to psychiatric disturbance. This may be attributable to organic brain syndrome secondary to multiple strokes, primary neuronal degeneration (Alzheimer's Disease) or other cause, or to longstanding pre-aged psychiatric illness such as manic-depressive illness, schizophrenia, or other psychiatric disorder (Miller & Barry, 1979). In addition to psychiatric problems the typical nursing home patient presents with concurrent involvement of multiple organ systems including chronic pulmonary edema, arthropathies, urologic disease, and neoplasms of various organs. The primary goal of the skilled nursing facility is to help residents to function to their maximal level physically, socially, and emotionally. In the long term setting, "care" takes precedence over "cure."

THE FAMILY

The nursing home also must strive for an effective working relationship with families of patients, for this is a vital element in a successful rehabilitation program. Unless family, patient, and nursing home agree on common goals for the patient, therapeutic programs will fail or be sabotaged. Tabak notes that family-patient relationships influence the quality of care in nursing homes (Tabak, 1978). The commandment to honor thy father and mother and the associated religious and cultural connotations cause some children who cannot personally care for their parents to become consumed with guilt. Therefore, nursing home placement almost uniformly is precipitated by a crisis situation; the old person may fall and break a hip, the long time companion may leave, the family caretaker may become ill. Goldfarb suggests that families often reject and delay institutionalization too long (Goldfarb, 1977).

The decision to admit the elderly parent into a nursing home can uncover and exacerbate unresolved family conflicts that have been dormant for decades (Kramer, 1976). Families who are guilt ridden about placing their parents in a nursing home often displace their guilt and scapegoat facts of the nursing home, commonly focusing on elements such as food. The professional staff must be trained to be able to differentiate between valid complaints about the dietary service and the use of food as a manifestation of psychological and/or other problems. Or the family member may preclude a therapeutic rehabilitation program by insisting that the patient "rest" in bed instead of participating in an ambulation retraining program. So common is family stress regarding nursing home placement that it is addressed in a new book, "designed to help families make the nursing home decision without guilt" (Manning, 1984).

Smith and Bengston found that nursing home placement of an elderly relative was not tantamount to family failure and breakdown but had the positive effect of renewing and enhancing family relationships (Smith & Bengston, 1979). In order to successfully care for the ill aged parent, the family too must be treated if orderly therapeutic patient-family goals are to be achieved (Miller, Bernstein, & Sharky, 1973). Families need counseling prior to admission in identifying their problems, help with separation and adaptation when the patient is in residence, and in many instances post discharge help to alleviate the pain of death.

THE THERAPEUTIC COMMUNITY

The therapeutic community is composed of the patient population, the physical environment, the interpersonal environment and the relationship of the interaction of patients, staff, families and the community on patient function. Since nursing is the largest and most central of all services provided in the nursing home, the quality of long term care is directly related to the medical leadership provided. By federal mandate in 1974, skilled nursing facilities participating in Medicare and Medicaid were required to retain a physician as medical director to coordinate medical services, to serve as liaison with attending physicians, and to evaluate professional and supportive staff services (U.S. Dept. HEW, Skilled Nursing Facilities, 1974). Medical direction legislation came about as a result of the deficits uncovered by former Senator Frank Moss and other nursing home critics in the early 70s (Subcommittee on Long Term Care of the Special Committee on Aging, 1975). Physician disinterest in the care of the chronically ill aged is in the process of changing. Medical schools are awakening to their responsibilities and are incorporating geriatrics into their curricula. In addition to diagnosis, geriatricians are being trained to manage and treat patients and to function as leaders of the clinical team, not as solo practitioners caring for individual patients (Miller, 1974).

In place of the general medical supervision given in the acute hospital, less frequent medical visits have put the nursing home director of nursing in the hub of almost all patient activities, including physical and occupational therapy, activities, nutrition, and social work. Because of the absence of immediate access to medical leadership, nursing diagnosis and knowledge of the clinical use and toxicology of commonly used drugs are essential tools of long term nursing. Most nursing home patients receive multiple drugs, females more than males. The average nursing home resident suffers from 3.9 conditions and data from a recent National Health Survey showed the average medications per patient amounted to 3.2 (National Health Survey Series, 1981).

All treating staff need to understand that body movement is crucial for the physical rehabilitation and emotional well being of the long term patient as well as to prevent disease and disability. For the intellectually impaired patient, nursing observation takes on an added dimension. Such persons often are unable to articulate symptoms. Thus nursing staff must be especially alert to subtle as well as overt cues: to smell, to touch, and to observation (Miller & Barry, 1979).

Both nurses and social workers become involved in family counseling in the long term care setting; nurses because of the infrequent physicians visits, and social workers to help the patient and family adjust to disability, separation, and to life in an institution.

While hospital dietetics are primarily technical in nature, in the skilled nursing facility meal times are social as well as nutritional experiences. When meal times, personal care, nursing, and rehabilitation therapies are completed, ample time is left to encourage patients to function socially in pursuit of a meaningful way of life. Successful recreation therapy where patients are stimulated to use their physical and mental capacities to the fullest prevents depression and psychological withdrawal so common in the nursing home setting (Miller & Barry, 1979).

EVALUATING A NURSING HOME

Much has been written on how to select a nursing home, including checklists prepared by periodicals and by agencies as diverse as the Public Health Service (U.S. Dept. HEW, Public Health Service,

1976), *The New York Times* (Brody, 1981), The American Medical Association (American Medical Association News Features, 1981), *Reader's Digest* (Ross, 1976), *Money Magazine* (Donnelly, 1975), The American Legion (Bradley, 1981) and the Union of American Hebrew Congregations (Shapiro). Although gerontologists and social workers espouse patient involvement in nursing home decision making, this is rarely feasible as most persons are admitted directly from the acute hospital setting—and more often family members are the decision makers and are directed to specific nursing homes by friends, social workers, neighbors, but rarely by physicians.

Meaningful evaluations of nursing homes by lay persons is extremely difficult. Untrained people tend to concentrate on the real estate, the colors, the presence or absence of odors, recreation programs, the food, whether residents "look happy." Certainly odors are not desirable but many intellectually impaired patients are incontinent and even with retraining programs will have accidents. And to expect residents to be happy and smiling when they have lost their health, their spouse, their home, may be unrealistic. Of more importance is the quality of medical and nursing care, the training of staff, the attitude of the treating staff. Much is written about the turnover of staff in nursing homes: Miller reports that staff remain in their positions in nursing homes primarily because of affection for their co-workers (Miller, Barry, & Ready 1976), emphasizing the need for congeniality amongst personnel as an essential component in staff recruitment.

Perhaps the most objective indicator of quality is "accreditation" proferred by the Joint Commission for Accreditation of Hospitals. Long term care facilities may voluntarily elect to participate in the accreditation process in their pursuit of quality. Unlike hospitals where "deemed status" results from accreditation (which means that hospitals are automatically certified for Medicare and Medicaid when they are accredited by the Joint Commission), long term care facilities are not eligible for deemed status and cannot be certified for Medicare and Medicaid even after being accredited by the Joint Commission.

Experienced nursing home administrators understand the relationship of size and increased depersonalization. Swedish nursing homes frequently are cited as models, and there, 70 beds are the preferred size (Kane & Kane, 1976). Curry and Ratliff (1973) and Townsend (1962) also equated smaller size with resident satisfaction. Ideally the long term care facility should be sufficiently large to provide all the necessary full time professional services but small enough so that a homeostasis may be developed between residents, families, and staff.

NON-INSTITUTIONAL LONG TERM CARE

Many factors have stimulated interest in the development of community based services for the frail elderly. Among these are demographic and deinstitutionalization pressures, more rigorous utilization review procedures currently related to D.R.G.s (diagnostic related groups) in the acute hospital, financial constraints of Medicare and Medicaid, and policy questions related to the appropriateness of institutional care, etc. Various solutions have been proposed related to care in the home for the chronic ill elderly.

Home care is not a new concept but long term home health care—known as the "nursing home without walls" concept in New York State—is receiving increasing attention (Miller, 1979). Conceptually any chronically disabled individual can remain at home if sufficient resources are expended and New York State is attempting to make long term home health care a viable alternative to nursing home care. The nursing home without walls requires that patients be given a choice between receiving long term health care at home or in an institution. Such programs are mandated to provide all the services available in a skilled nursing facility at approximately 75% of the per diem cost. Realistically, long term home health care can work only with the cooperation of an involved family, particularly when the patient is intellectually impaired. With the proper selection of candidates and a willing family support structure, long term home health care may prevent or, at a minimum, delay institutional care and provide a more humanistic solution to the plight of the ever increasing numbers of the ill aged. An inherent problem in this endeavor is the difficulty of supervising staff working alone in many settings throughout the community and maintaining quality (Miller, in press). Pegels commented on the need to control the expansion of services so as not to generate abuses which had occurred in the nursing home field (Pegels, 1980).

Respite Care

Shanas and Maddox noted that two or three times as many aged are homebound as in institutions, with the family the major caretaker (Shanas & Maddox, 1976). To enable families to continue to maintain their relative at home, respite care—an interval of rest or relief for the family—is receiving growing attention. Respite services can be provided in the home, freeing the family for brief excursions, or it may mean admitting the patient to a long term care facility for a time limited period when family is unable to provide the necessary support due to vacation, illness, or the like. Respite, like long term home health care, may preclude or delay nursing home admission. (See "Respite Care: Temporary Relief for Caregivers" by Jeanne E. Bader in this issue.)

THE FUTURE

Community based services for the ill elderly are certain to proliferate—including home care, day care, enriched housing, hospice care, comprehensive outpatient rehabilitation services, and other modalities yet to be developed. The so called "alternatives" really are not alternatives, for when long term inpatient care is required there is no alternative. As outreach options are promulgated and promoted, only the most disabled patient population with the least potential for rehabilitation will enter the nursing home. In effect, the nursing home of the future may look like a mausoleum and be even more repellent to patients and families who potentially need their services. Respite care probably will increase in usage as families learn how to spare themselves at specific intervals.

If long term institutions follow the hospital pattern, the number of free standing facilities is bound to diminish as nursing homes become part of multi-institutional systems. As the 450 teaching hospitals have been paradigms for 7,000 community hospitals, the teaching nursing homes espoused by Butler (Butler, 1981) can be models for over 18,000 nursing homes.

Finally, the most important component of long term care—the human resource component—will be better trained as medical, nursing, social work and other professional schools include gerontology and geriatrics in their curricula and offer students appropriate clinical experiences to enrich the didactic material. Interestingly, in a recent attitudinal study of first year medical students' response to nursing home exposure, only female students indicated interest in becoming geriatric physicians. Perhaps this is an indicator of the sex of future geriatric physicians (Miller & Lukashok, 1984). Women, of course, will continue to predominate in the long term care arena as frail elderly patients, as caretakers, and as health care workers. Whatever the model of care, the female influence cannot be underestimated.

REFERENCES

AMA offers pointers on how to pick a nursing home. (1981, August 18). *Medical Association News Features,* 1.

Bradley, J. (1981, January). A home for mama. *The American Legion, 110,* 14-15, 48-50.

Branch, L., & Jette, A. (1982). A prospective study of long term care institutionalization among the aged. *American Journal of Public Health, 72,* 1373-1379.

Brody, E., Johnson, P., Fulcomer, M., & Lang, A. (1983). Women's changing roles and help to elderly parents: Attitudes of three generations of women. *Journal of Gerontology, 38,* 597-607.

Brody, J. (1981, September 16). Selecting a nursing home. *New York Times,* Section C, 10.

Brotman, H. (1977). Life expectancy: Comparison of national levels in 1900 & 1974 and variations in state levels. *Gerontologist, 17,* 12-23.

Butler, R. (1981). The teaching nursing home. *Journal of the American Medical Association, 245,* 1435-1437.

Corman, J. (1976). Health services for the elderly. In B. Neugarten & R. Havighurst (Eds.). *Social policy, social ethics and the aging society* (pp. 81-88.) Washington D.C.: U.S. Gov't Printing Office.

Curry, R., & Ratliff, B. (1973). The effects of nursing home size on resident isolation and life satisfaction. *Gerontologist, 13,* 295-298.

Donnelly, C. (1975, October). A concerned relative's guide to old age care. *Money Magazine,* 77-86.

Goldfarb, A. (1977). Institutional care of the aged. In E.W. Busse & E. Pfeiffer. *Behavior and adaptation in late life* (pp. 264-292). Boston: Little, Brown & Co.

Health Care Financing Administration: Title XIX, grants to states for Medicaid Assistance programs (revised 1979, January). Washington, D.C., 2.

Kane, R., & Kane, R. (1976). *Long term care in six countries: Implications for the U.S.* Washington Fogerty International Center proceedings, Washington, D.C.: U.S. Gov't Printing Office.

Kastenbaum, R., & Candy, S. (1973). The 4% fallacy: A methodological empirical critique of extended care facility population statistics. *International Journal of Aging and Human Development, 4,* 15-21.

Keeler, E., Kane, R., & Soloman, D. (1981). Short and long term residents of nursing homes. *Medical Care, XIX,* 363-370.

Kramer, C. (1976). *Basic principals of long term care.* Springfield, Illinois: Charles C. Thomas.

Long Term Care Management. (1984, March 29). Washington, D.C., 3, 1-8.

Manning, D. (1984). *When love gets tough: The nursing home decision.* Hereford, Texas: In-Sight Books, Inc.

Miller, D. (1979). Nursing home without walls developed by New York State. *Hospitals, 53,* 44, 48.

Miller, D. (in press). Long term care and rehabilitation, In S. Wolfe (Ed.) *Handbook of health care services.* New York: McGraw-Hill.

Miller, D., & Barry, J. (1979). *Nursing home organization and operation.* Boston: C.B.I. Publishing.

Miller, D., Barry, J., & Ready, V. (1976). Staff turnover in long term care institutions. *Proceedings of the 2nd North American Symposium on Long Term Care Administration,* 129-154, Washington, D.C.: American College of Nursing Home Administrators.

Miller, D., & Lukashok, H. (1984). First year medical students' perceptions of aging and long term care. Manuscript submitted for publication.

Miller, M. (1974). Restructuring medical education for management of the chronically ill aged. *Journal of American Geriatrics Society, 22,* 501-510.

Miller, M., Bernstein, H., & Sharky, H. (1973). Denial of parental illness and maintenance of family homeostasis. *Journal of American Geriatrics Society, XXI,* 278-285.

National Health Survey Series. (1981, April). U.S. dept. of health and human services, Hyattsville, MA, *13.*

Pegels, C. (1980). Institutional versus non-institutional care of the elderly. *Journal of Health Politics, 5,* 205-212.

Ross, W. (1976, March). How to find a good nursing home. *Reader's Digest,* 91-95.

Shanas, E., & Maddox, G. (1976). Aging, health and organization of health resources. In R. Binstock & E. Shanas (Eds.). *Handbook of aging and the social sciences* (pp. 602-615). New York: Van Nostrand Reinhold Co.

Shapiro, S. (undated). Choosing a nursing home. *Committee on Aging Series,* New York: Union of American Hebrew Congregations.

Smith, L., & Bengston, V. (1979). Positive consequences of institutionalization: Solidarity between elderly parents and their middle aged children. *Gerontologist, 19,* 438-447.

Subcommittee on Long Term Care of the Special Committee on Aging, U.S. Senate. (1975). Doctors in nursing homes: The shunned responsibility. Washington, D.C.: U.S. Gov't Printing Office.

Tabak, H. (1978). The role of the family. *Journal of the American Health Care Association, 4,* 92-97.

Townsend, P. (1962). *The last refuge: A survey of residential institutions and homes for the aged in England and Wales.* London: Routledge and Kegan Paul.

U.S. Dept. HEW. (1974, October 3). Skilled nursing facilities, *Federal Register, 39,* 2238-2257.

U.S. Dept. HEW. (1976). *How to select a nursing home.* Washington, D.C.: Public Health Service Office of Nursing Home Affairs.

Respite Care:
Temporary Relief for Caregivers

Jeanne E. Bader, PhD

ABSTRACT. Recent respite care research is reviewed, advantages and disadvantages of respite- and home-based care are presented, and some recommendations are introduced. It may be more cost-effective to invest in caregivers' physical, financial, and emotional well-being than to provide the care required when caregivers become "patients." Practical and policy issues are raised regarding the desirability of investment in respite care.

Respite care is intended to provide temporary relief for caregivers of those who are unable to adequately care for themselves. Such caregiving is typically full-time, physically and emotionally exhausting, expected, and unappreciated by family, friends, and fellow taxpayers. In addition, such caregiving usually is long term and requires that the caregiver stay with the "patient" rather than work for pay. Furthermore, because private insurance plans provide little assistance to caregivers once the patient leaves the hospital, without externally supported programs all costs are out-of-pocket and may leave the caregiver destitute.

This paper will describe respite care, identify typical providers and beneficiaries of such care, and examine advantages and disadvantages of respite and home-based care. The paper will conclude with a discussion of practical and policy issues affecting provision of respite and home-based care.

FORMS OF RESPITE CARE

The simplest form of respite care is equivalent to babysitting—the services of an outsider to be physically present in the home while the caregiver takes a few hours away. When actual patient care is required while the caregiver is absent, more highly skilled paraprofessionals may be brought into the home. In-home services by home health nurses and professional (i.e., trained, salaried) homemakers may be required in more extreme situations. Placements in day care centers may provide daytime respite care as may temporary placements in foster homes. Finally, patients may be placed in institutional settings for a week or two, thereby permitting caregivers to take time off from caregiving—whether at home or on vacation.

PARTICIPANTS IN RESPITE CARE

The "Patients"

Among patients frequently requiring 24-hour caregiving are mentally retarded persons and those with developmental disabilities, cancer victims, and older persons (Project Share, 1981). The focus of this paper will be on respite care for families that include one or more older members in need of extensive care. Elderly respite care patients typically have multiple severe health problems, including rheumatoid arthritis and chronic organic brain syndrome as a result of stroke or Alzheimer's disease.

In the earliest stages of Alzheimer's Disease, for example, the victim is likely to retire "for health reasons." Not fully understanding what is happening, the patient may attempt to continue to function independently, using "aging" as an explanation for memory loss and cognitive dysfunction, physical deterioration, and social inappropriateness. As such symptoms accumulate and worsen, families may accelerate their efforts to understand, retard, or cope with the progress of the disease. Eventually, however, almost all families must seek assistance to supplement their own efforts in order to continue to function as a unit (Mace & Rabins, 1981). In particular, when it is the male head of household who is afflicted with Alzheimer's Disease, families may seek assistance with legal, financial, and health care matters that the victim of Alzheimer's Disease formerly handled for other family members (Glaze, 1982). Furthermore, families may be called upon to share decision making in new ways that require intergenerational respect and participation regarding the timing and course of family events (Archbold, 1980).

"Patients" whose caregivers may require respite care are frequently incontinent and may be abusive. Many experience sleep disturbances, eating disorders, and constipation, multiple sensory decrements (especially in hearing and vision), speech difficulties, and varying levels of disorientation to time, place, and person. They are unlikely to recognize the extent of caregiving provided for them and generally are unable to express appreciation for it or appropriate concern for the caregiver's physical, financial, or emotional well being.

Most older individuals requiring full time care are very old. This population, now know in the research literature as the old-old, comprises the fastest growing segment in U.S. society. The old-old population is expected to continue to expand well into the 21st century. Because it is this group who may be expected to have more—and more debilitating—chronic conditions, the need for caregiving and consequently for respite care will undoubtedly increase throughout the next fifty years.

The Caregivers

The primary beneficiaries of respite care are the caregivers. Such caregivers are twice as often women as men (i.e., older women caring for their husbands; and daughters and daughters-in-law caring for their mothers and mothers-in-law) (Colman, 1982; Fengler & Goodrich, 1979; Poulshock, 1982; Shanas, 1967; Silverman & Brache, 1979; Troll, 1971). One explanation for this imbalance is that most older men are married (75% in 1980) whereas most older women are widowed (52% in 1980). Lopata reports that 46% of the widows in her study (1973) had cared for their husbands at home before their deaths, 40% for more than one year. Also, the great majority of old people are women, thereby increasing the likelihood of women being both young-old caregivers and old-old care receivers. (There are 150 women 65 years of age or older for every 100 men 65 or older, 220 women 85 or older for every 100 men of the same age.) Each older caregiver, male or female, is also, of course, facing his or her own aging (Crossman, London, & Barry, 1981). Because of the increasingly disparate sex ratios among older U.S. citizens, because of the differences between older men's and women's marital statuses, and because of prevailing assumptions about "women's place" and their nurturing needs, females are more often the caregivers than men.

Respite Care Providers

Professionals and paraprofessionals providing respite care are also much more likely to be women than men. Given low pay, poor benefits, little chance for advancement, and societal assumptions that caregiving is "women's work," this is probably inevitable. One virtue of professional providers, besides the security caregivers feel leaving patients in their care, is that they can teach caregivers skills (e.g., prosthetic room design; how to transfer a person from bed to chair without injury). Skills training for caregivers continues to be rare and when it is available may require the caregiver to leave her home for a central location—something many caregivers are not willing to do.

The primary advantage of respite care for full time caregivers is that it provides welcome relief from caregiving—time to sleep, to take care of other business, or to attend a caregiver's training or support group (Gwyther, 1982; Mellor and Getzel, 1980, Weaver, 1982). Respite care makes possible long-term, home-delivered care. Health care providers will notice that many of the points made below also apply to adult day care, foster homes, and institutional placements.

ADVANTAGES AND DISADVANTAGES OF HOME-BASED CARE

It is frequently assumed that home-based care is superior in some way to institution-based care. It is said, for example, that families bring more affection, dignity, compassion, and patience—not to mention personalized care—to patient care than do institution personnel. The presumed superiority of in-home care is also based on the argument that "transfer trauma," expected with debilitated populations, can be avoided or postponed by avoiding or delaying relocation.

It is also asserted that it is the typical caregiver's preference to keep the patient at home rather than to institutionalize him or her (Poulshock, 1982; Wentzel, 1978). By providing respite care for the caregiver, it is further assumed that families (often lone individuals) will be able to provide care for years at a time. Though the research results are inconsistent (Congressional Budget Office, 1977; Eustis, Greenberg, & Patten, 1984), policy makers appear convinced that in-home care is less expensive for taxpayers (though not necessarily for the caregiver) than institutional care—at least in the short run.

While one might shy away from suggesting that there are disadvantages to home-based care for the patient, there are clearly enormous costs—and risks—to the caregiver of maintaining mentally and/or physically disabled family members at home. For one thing, round-the-clock caregiving is likely to affect the caregiver's health (Reece, Walz, & Hageboeck, 1983) and emotional well being (Cantor, 1983). Should the caregiver's physical and emotional health deteriorate, taxpayers may be asked to pick up the costs of care for the caregiver as well as the patient. Such hidden long-term costs have not yet been demonstrated because the longitudinal research necessary to examine such long term societal costs has not yet been done.

Another cost for the caregiver is social. At the very least, caregivers' privacy disappears and their social lives almost always suffer. At worst, feelings of abandonment, entrapment, and social isolation may ensue (Lezak, 1978; Worcester & Quayhagen, 1983). In fact, studies demonstrate that the level of informal support available to the caregiver (rather than patient characteristics) predict a caregiver's ability to continue in that role for extended periods of time (Fengler & Goodrich, 1979; Zarit, Reever, & Bach-Peterson, 1980).

A third cost for the caregiver is economic. Prolonged caregiving whether at home or elsewhere, is expensive. In fact, however, economic distress may both cause and result from the exigencies of caregiving. For example, at the very time that women are choosing (or finding it economically essential) to enter the paid labor force, the probability of their being called upon to become full-time caregivers is accelerating (Brody, 1981). It is precisely because of the economic realities of aging that some attorneys recommend that caregivers divorce their spouses in order to preserve at least a portion of their incomes for living expenses. Failure to do so, they say, may result in financial ruin, especially for aging women.

Another disadvantage of home-care by spouses is the deterioration that may occur in the affectional relationship between caregiver and patient, especially when they are husband and wife (Horowitz & Shindelmen, 1981). When husbands become the caregivers, the demands of role reversal may hasten that deterioration (Cantor, 1983).

Some families may be incapable of providing adequate care to dependent family members. The result may be neglect or even abuse of the individual (Hickey & Douglass, 1981). In such cases, professional assessments of patient needs may take precedence over family wishes. Institutionalization or foster home care may prove better than home-based care in such instances.

PRACTICAL CONSIDERATIONS

Can families do more than they are already doing for family members in need? Numerous studies have demonstrated that families overwhelmingly continue to be involved in caregiving for their older members, resorting to institutionalization only as a last resort (Brody & Gummer, 1967; Brody, 1966; Goldfarb, 1965; Townsend, 1965). For example, it has repeatedly been shown that 80% of the medically related home care provided to older people (e.g., injections, bandage change) is provided by their families (U.S. Public Health Service, 1972). Furthermore 97% of personal care services such as help with dressing, bathing, feeding, and toileting are provided by family and friends (White House Conference on Aging, 1981). When one considers that more then 50 percent of older persons claim to need such assistance (termed "personal care") with four or more personal care tasks, that amount of caregiving is extraordinary. These numbers take on added significance when it is recalled that failure to adequately accomplish one's "activities of daily living" (ADLs) is likely to cause the public to commit a person to an institution faster than the fact that their behavior is eccentric or bizarre (Lowenthal, 1964). Since patients whose caregivers desperately need respite care are typically more debilitated than those requiring help with ADLs alone, respite care may prove to be an inexpensive investment in the quality of care for all elders in need and in the prevention of "burn out" among most caregivers.

There are ways in which family members can "do more." They can take better care of one another. They can discuss openly and share some responsibility for the needs of the patient and the caregiver. And they can support one another when *none* of the options available to the caregiver appears to be guilt-free, adequate, or desirable (Roozman-Weigensberg & Fox, 1979; Rueveni, 1979). Fourth, they can recognize competing demands on the caregiver and on the family as a whole for what they are—demands for attention, energy, money, or support that may tax or exceed family members' patience or ability to respond in the desired way (Schmidt, 1980).

Not all families are willing to assume responsibility for dependent family members (Hanson, Sauer, & Seelbach, 1983). Some family members cannot bear to watch loved ones deteriorate. Others may foresee a dismal future for themselves as a parent declines. Age, education, income, living arrangements, and ethnicity also affect the extent to which families are willing and/or able to provide long term care (Adams, 1980; Brody, Poulshock, & Masciocci, 1978; Hanson, Sauer, & Seelbach, 1983; Ikegami, 1982; Krishef & Yoelin, 1981; Stoller & Earl, 1983; Shanas, 1979). The marital relations of "women in the middle" are particularly strained by the need to care for both younger and older family members (Cicirelli, 1983; Lang & Brody, 1983). Identifying professionals and para-professionals to do work of caregiving may prove difficult. Not only the demanding nature of full-time caregiving, but also its unrelenting (24-hour), often unappealing nature detract from recruiting possibilities—especially since the pay is low in comparison to salaries paid for more attractive positions. Other staffing considerations include how to assess respite care worker competence and reliability and how to cope with worker absenteeism and turn over.

POLICY ISSUES

States considering legislation regarding respite care will be interested in one of the findings of recent research: many respite care clients and their families rarely use community-based (i.e., "formal") services. While relevant data (from Washington and New York states) are only now emerging, the possible implications for designing funding packages are obvious: clients new to the services system would not necessarily "save" public dollars by choosing home-based services over institutional care. Why? Either because they would begin to use community-based services that they had, for whatever reason, not used before or because they would simply be delaying institutionalization of the "patient" at the expense of increasing the risk of need for care for themselves.

Federal Initiatives

Federal agencies variously label those older persons most in need of some form of long term care. Among those labels used are "the chronically impaired elders" (Administration on Aging), "the frail elderly" (Federal Council on Aging), and "the old-old" (U.S. House of Representatives Select Committee on Aging). Such persons are generally assumed to be at least 75 years of age and to show evidence of one or more chronic disabilities (health impairments or sensory decrements) that significantly affect overall functioning (e.g., by limiting mobility).

What have been the primary federal responses to an aging society? The first major federal response to the ongoing expansion of the old-old population was the enactment of Medicare and Medicaid. The boom in the nursing home "industry" that followed passage in 1965 of Titles XVIII (Medicare) and XIX (Medicaid) of the Social Security Act was immediate and continues in some locations to this day. Also in 1965 as federal policy expanded to include taxpayer support of institutional care for older and disabled persons, legislation was passed to create "information and referral" and nutrition programs for older Americans. This legislation, known as the Older Americans Act of 1965, has since been amended to place increasing emphasis on creating a comprehensive, coordinated approach to services provision for older persons—an approach that promotes area-wide (i.e., local) planning; targeting services to the poor, disabled, and minority subpopulations; and active involvement in decision making of older Americans. While the Act falls short of meeting its stated objectives (Crystal, 1982; Estes, 1979; Estes & Newcomer, 1983; Hudson, 1981) such policies nonetheless reflect federal willingness to sponsor some old age-specific services with tax funds.

Medicare, Medicaid, and Older Americans Act recognize the essential role of self-help and of "informal caregivers" (i.e., family, friends, neighbors). As pressure mounts to respond efficiently and at minimum cost to the growing needs of an increasingly aged population, new federal legislation might be expected to emerge to support both new models of financing long term care (e.g., diagnosis related groups [DRGs] and cash or tax incentives for home-based care) (Crowley, 1981). Current initiatives favor these and other massive cost-cutting measures, principally in Titles XVIII and XIX (Storey, 1983). Virtually all current federal initiatives seek to restrict eligibility for publicly financed services to persons most in need of them.

State Initiatives

Although a relatively recent development, respite care has been modestly supported by Medicaid and various state governments largely because it is believed to be a low cost way to keep chronically impaired persons out of costly institutions and because it is believed to be a low cost investment in the health of caregivers. Both arguments are essentially economic. While some states have used only state funds to support respite care (Connecticut, Louisiana), others have relied exclusively on federal programs (especially Titles XIX and XX of the Social Security Act) to support respite care (Kansas, Kentucky, Missouri). Still other states have mixed federal and state funds for the purpose (Delaware, Florida, Minnesota, Montana, New York, Vermont). (See Meltzer, 1982.)

Medicaid eligibility is required to receive respite care in some states (Florida, Kansas, Kentucky, Missouri). Kansas requires that community-based services in the area requesting respite care cost ten percent less than nursing home care in the same area. Some states rely to some extent on federally supported ACTION programs to provide volunteer staff for their respite care programs (Delaware, Vermont). Some states serve only persons over 60 or 65 years of age (Florida, Minnesota, Missouri). Kansas, Kentucky, Minnesota, and Missouri require "pre-admission screening" by a team of professionals before declaring new clients eligible for institution- or community-based services.

Colman (1982) points out that California denies in-home services to families with an "able and available spouse," thereby preventing her from earning an income *and* from receiving assistance with caregiving. Well-conceived respite care legislation is currently pending in California.

Four states passed respite care legislation in 1983. New Jersey and Illinois established respite care demonstration projects. Connecticut clarified its definition of respite care. And Texas introduced concurrent resolutions in support of the concept of respite care.

Also during 1983, several states (about one in four) applied for Medicaid waivers under Section 2176 of the federal Omnibus Budget Reconciliation Act of 1981 (PL-97-35). Such waivers permit Medicaid coverage of noninstitutional long-term care services for persons who are eligible for Medicaid and who would otherwise require an intermediate (ICF) or skilled (SNF) level of care. Foremost among these were waiver requests in support of case management. Respite care support was next most frequently requested (Intergovernmental Health Policy Program, 1984).

Other Initiatives

The national Older Women's League (OWL) designated expansion of respite care as one of its key objectives. In addition, OWL has recommended principles that "should be incorporated into reform of long term policy:

1. Caregivers' needs should be recognized through provision of adequate community services, including day care for disabled spouses.
2. Allocations should be made on the level of functional disability rather than on arbitrary means-tested eligibility requirements.
3. Incentives should be available for caregivers to facilitate home care.
4. Families and government should be seen as partners, not adversaries. Government supported services should supplement spousal care and should not be withdrawn when a wife is present.
5. The importance of support groups should be stressed. They serve as emotional support and as a focal point for advocacy initiatives.
6. In order to mitigate the pressures and pain of the caregiving spouse, there must be adequate support in all the areas of need—financial, physical, and emotional.'' (Colman, 1982, p. 11)

In order to promote these objectives, the Older Women's League has prepared model state-level legislation for use by its local chapters.

Other ideas that might be offered for consideration include the following:

1. Think of respite care as low-cost investment with very high pay off.
2. Encourage skills training and fitness programs with special emphasis on providing weight training for respite care providers and caregivers.
3. Develop interpersonal skills and, if necessary, programs to minimize the isolation and loneliness experienced by many caregivers.
4. Strengthen homemaker/home health services and their integration in support of individual families.
5. Extend respite care to foster care providers.
6. Collect longitudinal data on the effects of long term care on all the participants in the caregiving setting.
7. Encourage employers to accommodate the needs of caregivers for irregular hours and for emergency leaves.
8. Accelerate planning efforts for the graying of society and ask

the hard questions that need to be addressed regarding who the real client is, who should pay, and who should decide.
9. Reduce the emphasis on "innovativeness" as a criterion for public support. Several apparently successful programs have not been adequately evaluated to permit generalizations regarding cost/effectiveness/efficiency comparisons.
10. Allow caregivers to express their inevitable and appropriate feelings of grief and anger. For instance, avoid cutting off crying by hugging the caregiver too soon, or by saying "I know. I know."
11. Appreciate the caregivers.

As a life long activist and former caregiver for her physician husband, Janet Neuman observed her own need for relief from caregiving. Ten years ago, in her late eighties, she penned the following reflections.

DAY BY DAY

People do what they must do

A laugh will mask the hidden cry,
The need to walk when one would fly,
Tasks beckon when one would dream,
A sigh escapes to hide a scream.

While earth bound needs
Enslave a soul
Delay Obscures
The distant goal.

Along the road
A rose delights the eye;
A sparkling dew drop
Bright and gay
Eases the way, as
Day by day
People do what they must do.

Janet N. Neuman
Today, Tomorrow and Yesterday, 1978

The poem speaks of duty, hidden feelings, and suppressed needs.

Respite care enables women caretakers to meet some of their own needs as well as those of the people they care for. As such, respite care is a concept that deserves the support of feminists interested in women's health.

REFERENCES

Adams, J.P., Jr. (1980). Service arrangements preferred by minority elderly: A cross-cultural survey. *Journal of Gerontology Social Work, 3* (2), 39-57.

Archbold, P. (1980). Impact of parent caring on middle aged offspring. *Journal of Gerontological Nursing, 6* (2), 79.

Brody, E.M. (1981). "Women in the middle" and family help to older people. *The Gerontologist, 21* (5), 471-480.

Brody, E.M. (1966). The impaired elderly: A follow-up study of applicants rejected by a voluntary home. *Journal of the American Geriatrics Society, 14* (4), 414-420.

Brody, E.M., & Gummer, B. (1967). Aged applicants and non-applicants to a voluntary home: An exploratory comparison. *The Gerontologist, 7* (4), 234-243.

Brody, S.J., Poulshock, S.W., & Masciocci, C.F. (1978). The family caring unit: A major consideration in the long-term support system. *The Gerontologist, 18* (6), 556-561.

Cantor, M.H. (1983). Strain among caregivers: A study of experience in the United States. *The Gerontologist, 23* (6), 597-604.

Congressional Budget Office. (1977). *Long-term care for the elderly and disabled.* Washington, DC.

Circirelli, V.G. (1983). A comparison of helping behavior to elderly parents of adult children with intact and disrupted marriages. *The Gerontologist, 23* (6), 619-625.

Colman, V. (1982). *Till death do us part: Caregiving wives of severely disabled husbands.* Washington, DC: Older Women's League.

Crossman, L., London, C., & Barry, C. (1981). Older women caring for disabled spouses: A model for supportive services. *The Gerontologist, 21* (5), 464-470.

Crowley, D. (1981). Friends welcome. *Social Work Today, 13* (2), 16.

Crystal, S. (1982). *America's old age crisis: Public policy and the two worlds of aging.* New York, NY: Basic Books.

Estes, C.L. (1979). *The aging enterprise.* San Francisco, CA: Jossey-Bass.

Estes, C.L., & Newcomer, R.J. (1983). *Fiscal austerity and aging: Shifting government responsibility for the elderly.* Beverly Hills, CA: Sage.

Eustis, N., Greenberg, J., & Patten, S. (1984). *Long-term care for older persons: A policy perspective.* Monterey, CA: Brooks-Cole.

Fengler, A.P., & Goodrich, N. (1979). Wives of elderly disabled men: The hidden patients. *The Gerontologist, 19* (2), 175-183.

Glaze, B. (1982, Fall). A never-ending funeral: One family's struggle. *Generations,* 41.

Goldfarb, A.I. (1965). Psychodynamics and the three generation family. In E. Shanas & G.F. Streib (Eds.), *Social structure and the family: Generational relations* (pp. 10-45). Englewood Cliffs, NJ: Prentice Hall.

Gwyther, L.P. (1982, Fall). Caregiver self-help groups: Roles for professionals. *Generations,* 37-38.

Hanson, S.L., Sauer, W.J., & Seelback, W.C. (1983). Racial and cohort variations in filial responsibility norms. *The Gerontologist, 23* (6), 626-631.

Hickey, T., & Douglass, R.L. (1981). Neglect and abuse of older family members: Professionals' perspectives and case experiences. *The Gerontologist, 21* (2), 171-176.

Horowitz, A., & Shindleman, L.W. (1981). *Reciprocity and affection: Past influences on current caregiving.* Paper presented at meeting of the Gerontological Society of America, Toronto, Canada.

Hudson, R.B. (1981). *The aging in politics: Process and policy.* Springfield, IL: Charles C. Thomas.

Ikegami, N. (1982). Institutionalized and the non-institutionalized elderly. *Social Science and Medicine, 16* (23), 2001-2008.

Intergovernmental Health Policy Project. (1984). *Survey of Recent and Proposed Changes in State Medicaid Programs.* Washington, DC.

Krishef, C.H., & Yoelin, M.L. (1981). Differential use of informal and formal helping networks among rural elderly black and white Floridians. *Journal of Gerontological Social Work, 3* (3), 45-59.

Lang, A.M., & Brody, E.M. (1983). Characteristics of middle-aged daughters and help to their elderly mothers. *Journal of Marriage and the Family, 45* (1), 193-202.

Lezak, M.D. (1978). Living with characterologically altered brain injured patient. *Journal of Clinical Psychiatry, 39* (7), 592-598.

Lowenthal, M.F. (1964). *Lives in distress.* New York, NY: Basic.

Mace, N.L., & Rabins, P.V. (1981). *The 36-hour day. A family guide for persons with Alzheimer's Disease, related dementing illnesses, and memory loss in later life.* Baltimore, MD: Johns Hopkins University.

Mellor, J., & Getzel, G.S. (1980). *Stress and service needs of those who care for the aged.* Paper presented at the meeting of the Gerontological Society, San Diego, CA.

Meltzer, J.W. (1982). *Respite care: An emerging support service.* Washington, DC: The Center for the Study of Social Policy. Unpublished manuscript.

Poulshock, S.W. (1982). *The effects on families of caring for impaired elderly in residence.* Unpublished manuscript.

Project Share. (1981). *Human services bibliography series: Respite and crisis care.* Rockville, MD: National Clearinghouse for Improving the Management of Human Services.

Reece, D., Walz, T., & Hageboeck, H. (1983). Intergenerational care providers of non-institutionalized frail elderly: Characteristics and consequences. *Journal of Gerontological Social Work. 5* (3), 21-34.

Roozman-Weigensberg, C., & Fox, M. (1979). Groupwork approach with adult children of institutionalized elderly: An investment in the future. *Journal of Gerontological Social Work, 2* (4), 355-362.

Rueveni, U. (1979). *Networking families in crisis. Intervention strategies with families and social networks.* New York, NY: Human Sciences Press.

Schmidt, M.G. (1980). Failing parents, aging children. *Journal of Gerontological Social Work, 2* (3), 259-268.

Shanas, E. (1979). The family as a social support system in old age. *The Gerontologist, 19* (2), 169-174.

Silverman, A.G., & Brache, C.I. (1979). As parents grow older: An intervention model. *Journal of Gerontological Social Work, 2* (1), 77-85.

Stoller, E.P. & Earl, L.L. (1983). Help with activities of everyday life: Sources of support for the noninstitutionalized elderly. *The Gerontologist, 23* (1), 64-70.

Storey, J.R. (1983). *Older Americans in the Reagan era: Impacts of federal policy changes.* Washington, DC: The Urban Institute.

Townsend, P. (1965). The effects of family structure on the likelihood of admission to an institution in old age: The application of a general theory. In E. Shanas & G.F. Streib (Eds.), *Social structure and the family: Generational relations* (pp. 163-187). Englewood Cliffs, NJ: Prentice Hall.

Troll, L. (1971). The family of later life: A decade review. *Journal of Marriage and the Family, 33* (2), 263-290.

U.S. Public Health Service. (1972). Home care for persons 55 and over, United States: July 1966-June 1968. *Vital and Health Statistics, 10* (73).

Weaver, D.A. (1982, Fall). Tapping strength: A support group for children and grandchildren. *Generations,* 45.

Wentzel, M.L. (1978). Emotional considerations in the institutionalization of an aged parent. *Journal of Health and Human Resources Administration, 1,* 177-185.

White House Conference on Aging. (1981). *Chartbook on aging in America.* Washington, DC: U.S. Department of Health and Human Services.

Worcester, M.I., & Quayhagen, M.P. (1983). Correlates of caregiving satisfaction: Prerequisites to elder home care. *Research in Nursing and Health, 6* (2), 61-70.

Zarit, S.H., Reever, K.E., & Bach-Peterson, J. (1980). Relatives of the impaired elderly: Correlates of feelings of burden. *The Gerontologist, 20* (6), 649-655.

Alzheimer's Disease:
A Practical, Psychological Approach

Lenore S. Powell, EdD, NCPsyA

ABSTRACT. Alzheimer's Disease affects approximately two million people. It is a crippling, organic brain disorder that causes loss of recent memory, intellectual deterioration, unpredictable behavioral changes, and personality deterioration. The fourth leading cause of death among the elderly, it also affects younger people. The disease has two victims, the Alzheimer patient and the caregiver. Caregivers often experience shame, embarrassment, denial, frustration, anger, depression, and guilt as they care for an Alzheimer patient. This paper provides information about the disease and it's manifestations, along with practical suggestions to help both the Alzheimer patient and the caregiver.

Alzheimer's Disease, once called the "silent epidemic" is now the disease of the future because of the large number of people who will develop and die from it. Currently the fourth leading cause of death among the elderly (Raber, 1983), it also accounts for 75% of dementia in the elderly (Fryer, 1983). It affects between 5 and 10% of the population over the age of 65 and between 10 and 20% of those over the age of 75. At least 600,000 patients with Alzheimer's disease are currently in nursing homes and for every person in a nursing home there are 4 or 5 living in the community who are also affected (Eisdorfer & Cohen, 1982). The disease usually develops between the ages of 45 and 65, but the youngest person on record is 28 and it also affects the middle-aged. The illness reduces life span by about one-third. Its duration may be between 1 to 16 years with an average of 6 to 8 years. While more women seem to be affected than men (Kosick & Growdon, 1982) this may be due to women's greater longevity. Alzheimer's does not appear to be related to education, occupation, economic, or social status.

Autopsy is required for a definitive diagnosis but through the exclusion of a variety of other factors, such as metabolic disorder, toxic poisoning, other diseases, and depression, diagnosis can generally be made. Diagnosis is one of exclusion, made by screening symptoms that may be indicative of other illnesses. A battery of neurological, physical, and psychological examinations is used in determining whether Alzheimer's disease is the cause of the behavioral changes being seen in either an elderly or younger person.

SYMPTOMS

Alzheimer's Disease is technically described in the Diagnostic Manual of the APA (American Psychiatric Association, 1980) as Primary Degenerative Dementia, a dementia arising in the senium and presenium, often abbreviated as SDAT, Senile Dementia Alzheimer's Type. It was named for the German neurologist Alois Alzheimer who in 1906 described disease of middle age characterized by a progressive deterioration in behavior including jealousy and paranoid traits, in addition to memory and intellectual disturbances (Reisberg, 1981). Alzheimer believed that the dementia (loss of reason) as well as the microscopic lesions in the brain which characterized the disease were caused by arteriosclerosis. Thus it was believed that senility was caused by hardening of the arteries. Not until the 1960s did the autopsies of demented and non-demented patients show this was erroneous (Fishman, 1984). Since then other explanations of its origin have been sought.

Recent memory loss is the most prevalent symptom of Alzheimer's Disease. One tragedy of the illness is that without memory, time is a meaningless abstraction and every routine experience becomes a venture into the unknown. Loss of memory is a painful source of distress because without memory we don't know if we have loved or felt pleasure, sorrow, or regret. We also don't know if we are loved and our sense of security and reliability is so shaken that we become anxious and afraid even of those people on whom we once could depend. Both victims of the illness, the patient and the caregiver, feel alone, abandoned, and afraid.

FOUR PHASES OF ALZHEIMER'S

Although each case varies, there are four identifiable phases of the illness, each with its own set of symptoms. In the first phase of Alzheimer's disease, relatives are unsure that anything is wrong with the person. Since the onset is insidious, there may be less energy, drive and initiative, a slowness to react and to learn new things. In the beginning stages the person seeks and prefers familiar people, places, and things, avoids that which is unfamiliar, seems to be less discriminating, and becomes easily upset and angered, especially when words are lost. Clarisse Havemeyer tells about her father:

> Dad used to be champ at word games. He was a great reader and he loved crossword puzzles and the English language. One day we were talking about witchcraft, and he kept looking for a word to describe Satan. I came up with words like "devil, wicked." He said "Mephistophiles," but there was another word like devilish and he just couldn't think of it. He kept saying "dev-den." I couldn't think of it either. But Dad got so irritated that he stormed out of the room to the kitchen and barked at my mother, "Let's go home!" I never saw him so upset! Just over a word! I guess he meant "demonic"; I looked it up in Roget's Thesaurus and called to tell him, but he wouldn't come to the phone. Poor Dad!

Communication, comprehension, and word finding abilities break down. Difficulties in these aspects of abstract thinking and calculation indicate the development of a dementia that is progressive (Katzman, 1982).

The second phase of the illness brings more losses. The patient's speech slows. She may misunderstand what she hears, lose the thread of a story, or miss the punchline of a simple joke. She has difficulty sleeping, may be unable to calculate, and needs help with balancing the checkbook.

Planning ahead and making decisions becomes very troublesome, as it did for Mr. Skolnick. His daughter told us that the illness came on so gradually that she wasn't aware of it. They were partners in their grocery business, and she depended on him all the time. Suddenly he couldn't make decisions about how many cases of tuna or toilet paper to order. In the beginning, her father denied that there was any problem. When she finally realized something was wrong, she felt helpless and didn't know what to do.

Forgetfulness, inability to recognize familiar objects, places and people, sounds or words commonly increase. Agitation and confusion are seen in the day-night reversal known as the "sundowner syndrome'': the patient is active during the night but sleeps during the day. There is also perseveration: repetitive action and verbalization, i.e., asking the same questions repeatedly. Chewing and swallowing food become difficult and choking may ensue; there may be excessive interest in food or total disinterest. Becoming increasingly self-absorbed, the impaired person seems totally insensitive to the needs and feelings of others and seems to avoid any situations that may end in failure. The person in this phase continues to function, but may need supervision.

Obvious disability marks the third phase of the disease. The victim loses normal orientation to time and place and is not able to identify familiar people or events.

> My husband and I went to our grandson's birthday party. He didn't want to go, but I said ''We're going,'' and I didn't give him an alternative. At the party, he had fun, he laughed and joked; he has a terrific sense of humor, and he remembers things that happened years and years ago. He had a good time. On the way home he admitted that. The next day I mentioned some of the nice people that were at the party. He said, ''What party?'' I was stunned. I couldn't believe it. He had totally forgotten about the party as if he'd never been there.

As described by his wife, Mr. Kenyon is now very lethargic, invents words of his own, and needs repeated instruction and direction. Unsure of himself, he behaves in unexpected ways and expressed very little warmth to close friends and relatives. While memory of recent events fails, he seems to recall the past with astonishing clarity. There is a considerable change in his behavior, some of which is exaggerated and often bizarre.

The fourth phase of the illness finds the victim apathetic, unable to get around a familiar house or apartment, wandering, needing help with all of the activities that encompass daily life and self-care. There is continued loss of recent and remote memories; syllables, words, and phrases are repeated over and over. Failure to recognize oneself in the mirror, and inability to recognize other people is common. Also, in this phase depression, delusions or delirium may occur. With the gradual memory loss comes loss of personal dignity followed by lack of confidence.

In the last stage of Alzheimer's disease, the patient's disorientation is complete. Continued recent memory loss and past memories fade, gait disturbance, feebleness, incontinence, and no communication on a verbal level ensues.

Cause of Death

Alzheimer victims are susceptible to paralysis that is progressive and also to respiratory difficulties such as bronchopneumonia, infections, and kidney failure which usually are the major causes of death. Recently, however, death certificates have stated the cause of death as Alzheimer's Disease, demise of the brain which has prematurely aged and shriveled.

ETIOLOGY

Relatives of people with Alzheimer's disease are four times more likely to develop it than the general population (Gwyther & Matteson, 1983). Research indicates a higher risk if a parent or sibling was affected at an early age, although having a sibling who developed Alzheimer's disease after the age of 70 does not increase the risk (Butler & Emr, 1982). About 80% of siblings are expected to be free of dementia of Alzheimer's type at age 80 even if a brother or sister had the illness. Genetic predisposition to the disease does not necessarily mean that it will develop since such predispositions are modifiable (Matsuyuma & Jarvik, 1982).

Recent studies of a disease known as Scrapie and found in sheep and goats indicate a new possible cause of Alzheimer's Disease: prions, infectious agents that contain protein and little or no nucleic acid. The prions aggregate into long rods resembling the amyloid collections found in the brains of Alzheimer patients. The senile plaques of Alzheimer patients are composed of amyloid which was thought to be a waste product of the disease process. However, amyloid may be related to the cause of Alzheimer's disease (Prusiner & Bernheim, 1984). Thus, an infectious agent such as a virus which incubates for approximately 30 years may be the cause of Alzheimer's Disease. A diagnostic test is being worked on in the research laboratories of the University of California in San Diego that would detect substances in the blood that become amyloid fibers inside the blood vessels of the brain (Glenner, 1984). All of the new research is encouraging and may point the way to a cure for Alzheimer's Disease.

CARING FOR THE PATIENT
WITH ALZHEIMER'S DISEASE

Costs of Care

The financial cost of caring for Alzheimer disease patients is substantial; governmental costs for institutionalization of such patients are approximately $20 billion a year. By the year 2000 it is estimated that 4 million Americans will have this disease and that the cost of care will go up to $78 billion (Geriatrics Update, 1983). The financial burden to families who are providing most of the care to those living at home is gargantuan; just as important are the costs of devotion and courage, for the physical, social, and emotional burdens of love are essential and priceless.

Should Patients Be Told They Have Alzheimer's Disease?

In the mild or moderate stage of the illness Alzheimer patients may recognize, although be unable to explain, their own cognitive decline and difficulties. The caregiver must determine whether withholding information about the illness will increase anxiety and foster depression. Patients have the right to know but their capacity to understand and the inability to remember are also factors in disclosing information. Most caregivers feel impelled to be forthright and honest, sharing facts with the patient in an empathic manner. Early knowledge may permit the patient and the family to attend to financial planning, legal responsibility, power of attorney, etc. It allows time to mourn and to prepare for the care of dependent spouses and children. At this point the family should begin to develop a support system that may include a self-help group, a home health aide, physician, attorney, and psychotherapist to help them prepare for emotional, physical, and financial stress as the deterioration of the victim increases.

Living with Victims of Alzheimer's Disease

The burden of love is living with the helpless and knowing they cannot be spared the pain of losing themselves; nor can caregivers be spared the pain of their losses. Indeed, our feelings influence the way we treat our patients and also how we treat ourselves. When an individual is no longer intellectually vigorous and can no longer learn, think, or remember, it is important to investigate the causes of these events. Memory loss can be a symptom of a number of treatable illnesses, including depression. However, when recent memory fails (that is, one can no longer remember where they live or how to get there, time is meaningless, numbers no longer significant, and familiar people are strange), and when this is accompanied by disorientation, confusion, and behavioral changes, Alzheimer's Disease must be considered (Powell & Courtice, 1983). Once acknowledged, the fears of "How will I take care of her?" or "Will I inherit the disease from my father?", arise. The pain of knowing that there is no known cause and no known cure leads to enormous frustration. Frustration turns into anger when Pop repeats the same sentences over and over again or when Mom seems to act silly by asking "When do we eat?" after having just had a sumptuous meal or when she wants to leave as soon as the couple arrive at their daughter's home.

In everyday life with an Alzheimer patient, predictability is important. They need a structured environment that is secure and safe from physical harm. Familiarity is a source of comfort to the patient who becomes more confused in unfamiliar surroundings. An organized room and possessions, plus the labeling of objects that are used regularly, can be very helpful. Placing pictures of stored objects on cabinets is useful. For example, a picture of a pair of socks in the drawer where socks are kept. Also useful are lists as reminders of tasks to be done.

Giving answers to questions patients ask is a way of accepting the fact that a relative is no longer capable of carrying out the ordinary business of daily living as she has done for a lifetime. She is not being willful, stubborn, obstinate, or deliberately destructive, but simply no longer has the capacities that all of us take for granted. Simplifying and being consistent with her is extremely important. Caregivers must learn to check their own fears when an Alzheimer patient has a "catastrophic reaction," which includes outbursts of rage or continual crying. The caregiver must treat the patient gently and then deal with their own feelings of frustration and sadness by talking to a friend, meditating, getting some physical exercise, or perhaps professional counseling.

Needs of the Caregiver

The emotions of the caregiver range from denial to shame, embarrassment, fear and frustration; from anger to depression and guilt. Relatives may feel shame and embarrassment over inappropriate behavior such as shoplifting or sexual exhibitionism. The caregiver's mortification at the victim's behavior leads to frustration, agitation and anger. Also, the caregiver's anxieties about their own lives and the extraordinary responsibilities caring for such a person engenders may produce irritation at nurses and physicians who don't have the much desired answers.

Understanding anger as a reaction to frustration is important and may enable the caregiver to deal with the situation in more adaptive and appropriate way—this includes counting to ten or polishing floors or hitting tennis balls. Minimizing frustration via the physical release of energy is an effective way of letting off steam. Using visual imagery such as imagining a peaceful scene that feels relaxing can calm down an irritated caregiver. Getting away for an hour or sharing feelings with a confidant is the best way to deal with angry feelings. Talking things out with someone who will listen empathically helps the angry person to feel understood. As she discovers she has control, self-confidence returns and feelings of self-esteem rise.

Anger is a constructive force that mobilizes caregivers to protect and assert themselves when it is necessary and appropriate to do so. However, when they show anger towards a beloved parent or spouse with Alzheimer's disease, in response to actions they are no longer able to control, and for which they are therefore no longer accountable, then anger is being used destructively. Some caregivers become self-destructive and wind up hating themselves for their behavior. They also limit their capacity to help the patient when anger replaces the loving feelings of the past. The daily routines of feeding, bathing, dressing, and constant watchfulness then become even more frustrating and exhausting. Caregivers feel guilty when they are out of control. Thus it is important for the psychotherapist to help them interrupt the vicious circle of anger/blow-up/guilt/more anger. Understanding anger as a voluntary response (a way in which she decides to express her frustration, rather than as something that just happens to her) may enable her to do something about it. Caregivers can learn to manage and use their anger in the interest of their survival as loving and effective caregivers. However, to do so they must first decide to take care of their own needs and understand and be compassionate to their own emotions.

Both the Alzheimer patient and the caregiver may be depressed. For the patient it is extremely important that there be a differential diagnosis between dementia and depression, since depression *can* be treated.

When caregivers, driven by feelings of devotion and duty, exceed their own physical and emotional capacities, they may become clinically depressed. Caregivers sometimes feel like "married widows or widowers." They react to the impact of being deprived of a formerly loving, nurturing and responsive parent or spouse with grief; they begin to prematurely mourn the loss of the beloved and the experience of loss may lead to a reactive depression. Psychotherapists can help caregivers to tolerate feelings of sorrow and their sense of loss. With professional counseling, the caregiver will be helped to acknowledge that the loved one has changed. It is sound advice to the caregiver to acknowledge the change and take one day at a time. Patients and caregivers should try to derive satisfaction from small, immediate pleasures. This mitigates the long term view of the realistic limitations on their lives. Sharing feelings with close friends and relatives or with other caregivers in a psychotherapy group is also very helpful for the depressed person, especially when expressions of empathy are offered. However, Alzheimer support groups that are not professionally led may not be able to mobilize the depressed caregiver's resources.

Someone who is frightened to be alone and preoccupied with thoughts of their own death is at risk and must be treated by a competent psychotherapist who knows how to help them through their despair. The depressed caregiver who feels guilty and locks guilt away needs a place to release these powerful feelings through the catharsis of psychotherapy. Even though depressions are cyclical and patients feel better in time, immediate treatment by a competent psychotherapist provides the support, encouragement, understanding and availability of an empathic ear that is necessary in treating depression.

Feelings of guilt may also trouble caregivers. Conscience helps us to feel good about ourselves when we are in harmony with our own and society's values. However, when a caregiver behaves selfishly, or thinks they are, they may inflict the punishment of guilt upon themselves. Sometimes caregivers experience pangs of guilt over things they knowingly ignore in their patients. They may also feel guilt over making errors in treating the patient or their own indiscretions. Caregivers may be guilty of losing control over their emotions, for example when they become angry with the Alzheimer patient for repeating things again and again; or when the constant frustration of tending to her needs causes them to abuse the patient. However, when the caregiver feels guilty about things that aren't in his/her power to control, the unconscious is taking over. Guilt over institutionalizing a relative is the most difficult feeling to dissipate and usually professional intervention is the only way to work through these feelings. The therapist must be aware that often guilt feelings are tied to unconscious wishes and have genetic roots. Thus, this aspect of the treatment takes time. Helping the caregiver to talk about guilty feelings can be extremely helpful in permanently relieving the burden of that uncomfortable emotion and in assisting the caregiver with painful decisions.

Those who deal with Alzheimer's disease must recognize that both the patient and the caregiver are victims and that adequate treatment is needed by both. Help should be offered in practical terms, enlisting as wide a support network as possible.

REFERENCES

American Psychiatric Association. (1980). *Quick reference to the diagnostic criteria from DSM III*, 66.

Butler, R.N., & Emr, M. (1982). SDAT research: Current trends. *Generations, 7*(2), 17.

Eisdorfer, C., & Cohen D. (1982, Fall). Health policy implications: Risking a serious crisis. *Generations, 7*(1), 36.

Fischman, J. (1984). The mystery of Alzheimer's. *Psychology Today, 27.*

Fryer, D.G. (1983, Summer). Dementia in the elderly. *Bulletin of the Mason Clinic, 37*(2), 67.

Geriatrics Update. (1983, Nov/Dec). *Geriatric Consultant, 99.*

Glenner, J. (1984, May 16). *Biochemical & Biophysical Research Communications.*

Gwyther, L.P., & Matteson, M.A. (1983). Care for the caregivers. *Journal of Gerontological Nursing, 9*(2), 93.

Katzman, R. (1982, Fall). The complex problems of diagnosis. *Generations, 7*(1), 11-13.

Kosick, K., & Growdon, J.H. (1982). Aging, memory loss and dementia. *Psychosomatics, 23*(7), 746.

Matsuyuma, S.S., & Jarvik, L.F. (1982, Fall). Genetics: What the practitioner needs to know. *Generations, 7*(1), 19.

Powell, L.S., & Courtice, K. (1983). *Alzheimer's disease: A guide for families.* Massachusetts: Addison-Wesley.

Prusiner, S.B., & Benheim, P.E. (1984, Spring). Creutzfeldt-Jakob disease—A related disorder. *ADRDA Newsletter, 4*(1), 6.

Raber, P. (1983). The dementia dilemma. *Geriatrics, 38*(8), 121.

Reisberg, B. (1981). *Brain failure.* New York: Free Press.

Reproductive Cancer

William J. Mann, MD, FACOG

ABSTRACT. The increasing life expectancy of our population will mean that by the year 2000 we may expect a large number of women to be in age groups at significant risk for malignancies of the female reproductive tract. It is very unlikely that we will soon understand the cause of cancer, and effective new therapies are not to be anticipated. Rather, improved survival and diminished morbidity must be obtained by insuring ready and equal access to state of the art treatment, for the patient and physician.

By calendar year 2000, over 12% of the population will be over the age of 65, and more than half of these individuals will be female. Thus, we will have a large population of elderly females, a population in whom the incidence of carcinomas of the reproductive tract is at its peak. The sixties is the decade in which the gynecologic malignancies peak in incidence—cancer of the cervix, cancer of the endometrium and cancer of the ovary are all diseases of the aging female. If one looks at the ten leading causes of death, cancer is first for females age 35 to 54, second for ages 55 to 74, and third for ages 75 and older. We are looking then to a century which will be heralded by a predictable increase in cancers of the female reproductive organs (Silverberg & Lubera, 1983).

Facing this bleak prospect, we may consider two aspects: the attitude and understanding of the lay community, and the aggressiveness and success of the medical profession. In the essay, *Illness as Metaphor*, Susan Sontag points out that while tuberculosis was the dreaded disease that carried a social stigma in the past, cancer has replaced it as the metaphor of uncleanliness—the body rotting from within (Sontag, 1978). Fortunately, we have seen a rise in awareness and compassion in the paramedical and behavioral sciences leading to a re-evaluation of the attitude of medical science toward cancer patients. While once it may have been thought that cancer was a cataclysmic diagnosis, leading to withdrawal from the mainstream of human life and rapid demise, it is now more accepted that cancer, in its many forms, is a chronic illness, which while debilitating, does not necessarily preclude the cancer victim from participating in the daily routine of productive life. Improved techniques of chemotherapy, radiotherapy, and surgery, as well as inventive combinations of these treatments, have led not only to more patients being cured, but also to many more patients being able to continue their daily routine with minimal disruption. What we must now seek is a sense of awakened appreciation for the chronicity of cancer, the pain and emotional cost of the disease to both the victim and the family, and the increasing sophistication of the medical armentarium which is used to fight malignancy. We have now reached a time when consumer awareness must be enthusiastically adopted by the cancer victim: however, quack remedies, shallow platitudes and faulty holistic concepts must be prevented from obscuring the benefits that can be obtained from aggressive chemotherapy, megavoltage radiotherapy, radical surgery, and multi-system whole body medical support. On the one hand, shoddy thinking and platitudes must be avoided, and on the other, excessive use of technology solely for the sake of technology itself must be decried.

CANCER OF THE BREAST

In reviewing the results in the past three decades of the management of cancer of the breast, we epitomize the dichotomy in thought which exists between the medical profession and the lay public. Here is a disease in which the relative five year survival in 1960-1963 was 63%, in 1970-1973 68%, and in 1973-1980 74%, and yet, we find wide-based general criticism of accepted cancer management (Henderson & Conellos, 1980). The problem here relates to the controversy over the use of radical mastectomy as opposed to less deforming and less radical therapy; notably the use of lesser surgical procedures and combined radiation therapy, or radiation therapy alone. In a sense, though, this controversy parallels the predicted situation for the other genital malignancies we will be discussing. The cure rate for most cancer of the reproductive organs has probably leveled off or been maximized. Currently acceptable techniques of treatment, i.e., surgery, radiation and chemotherapy, are being optimally utilized alone and in combination. We can therefore no longer focus on survival as the sole criteria by which to justify therapy. Rather, we must weigh the morbidity, cost (both emotional and financial), and the available alternatives.

For cancer of the breast, as well as other malignancies of the female reproductive organs, our only significant chance of improving survival lies in early diagnosis or prevention. Herein lies the crux of the problem. For carcinoma of the breast, we can create a typical patient profile, consisting of nulliparity, late first pregnancy and other factors, but then we are unable to take this clinical profile and effectively apply it to benefit a specific woman. Rather, we are left with the hopes of developing a mass screening technique which can, with minimal side effect or risk, select out those patients with early, nonmetastatic breast carcinoma. Mammography, ultrasonography, thermography, and now NMR scanning, have all been supported by their advocates as superior methods of screening for early disease, yet experts disagree as to which method is the most sensitive. Though mammography appears to have more advocates than other techniques, the question as to the true efficacy or benefit of these screening methods in preventing cancer or saving lives is unproven. In fact, these screening methods only seek out early cancer, and cannot be expected to prevent cancer: they can only be expected to find cancer in its earliest and most treatable and curable stages. When one complicates the picture by requiring the screening method used to be shown cost effective, or acceptable to a third party payer in terms of outlay of funds, a confusing situation becomes even more perplexing. Breast self-examination remains the best and proven means of detecting early lesions. It must be taught not only by physicians, but also as part of the high school health curriculum (Moskowitz, 1983).

It would appear that the combination of less radical surgery and radiation therapy may be as effective in curing cancer as the previously accepted radical surgical approach. However, decades of careful meticulous study will be required to confirm this opinion and even then the question of the side effects, toxicity and emotional stress of surgery and radiation compared to radical surgery will be difficult to evaluate. One must recognize that treatment failures, or recurrence of cancer, can occur five, ten, or even fifteen years after treatment.

In the next twenty years we may see increasing efforts to salvage patients who are now either incurable with current accepted treatment modalities, or whose survival is short. We will be trying to prolong survival, recognizing that cure is not possible, or we will be trying to minimize the toxicity and side effects of currently accepted treatments. These goals are not as desirable as determining the cause of breast cancer and effecting a cure by means of prevention. However, cancer is not one disease, but thousands of different diseases, and it is unlikely that they will all have a common pathway of development. Even if such a common pathway exists, there will be a myriad of ways to enter into it, and prevention will require blocking all of them. Therefore, cure or prevention for carcinoma of the breast (or any carcinoma which is not clearly linked to an environmental agent), is not likely to happen. We can anticipate better palliation, salvage of patients proven incurable, and use of less radical combined treatment modalities, which are less deforming and more emotionally and surgically acceptable to the patient. And we must do this while working under financial constraints, which, by definition, are not considerate of the suffering of patients.

CARCINOMA OF THE CERVIX

The adoption of the Papanicolaou smear, a rapid, inexpensive and safe screening method, has led to an increasing frequency of diagnosis of premalignant lesions of the cervix and thus prevented cervical malignancies. Simultaneously, the development of radical pelvic surgery and of radical pelvic irradiation, has led to an improved and increased cure rate for frankly invasive cervical carcinomas. Numerous large etiologic studies documented the risk factors for cancer of the cervix, i.e., multiple sexual partners, early age of intercourse, multiple births. However, it would appear that the limits of radical surgery have been reached, and that the complication rate has now been reduced to a minimum, less than 1%, and the cure rate taken to a maximum, greater than 85%. Similarly, radical irradiation of the pelvis has yielded comparable cure rates, and while the complication rate of 3-5% remains, surgical or medical correction of complications is readily available. Multiple attempts to combine the two modalities have not yielded an improved survival but have increased the complication rate experienced by the patients (Morrow & Townsend, 1981). It is not likely that we can look to either surgery, radiation, or a combination of the two modalities to improve survival in the future for patients with carcinoma of the cervix.

Risk factors help in selecting out the population in whom screening may yield a high result of preinvasive disease. However, with any one individual patient, recognition of risk factors is of no help and only individualized treatment can be used. Thus, while we understand the various patients at risk, and even recognize the possible relationship of the papilloma virum to the etiology of carcinoma of the cervix, this information currently helps us not at all in managing the individual patients in a preventative manner. All we can offer is screening of high risk populations, and ablation of preinvasive lesions when they are diagnosed.

Currently, screening is accomplished by the Papanicolaou smear, and the acceptance of colposcopy, that is visualizing the cervix with a microscope, on an outpatient basis. Colposcopically directed biopsy will then allow the establishment of a diagnosis, and in the majority of cases the lesion can be treated in an outpatient setting using cryosurgery, laser surgery, or simple excision. Operative removal of the lesion, the so-called cervical cone, can now be avoided in over 90% of patients, and rarely if ever is hysterectomy indicated for destruction of these preinvasive lesions.

When a frankly invasive cancer is found, surgery or radiation can be offered with a reasonable hope of complete cure, depending on the stage of disease at the time of diagnosis. Hysterectomy consists of removal of the uterus, and the radical hysterectomy which is used in treatment for carcinoma of the cervix, consists of not only removal of the uterus but also removal of the supporting tissues or connective tissues surrounding the uterus and also the lymph nodes of the pelvis. The ovaries are not removed, routinely, as part of a radical hysterectomy. Should this surgery be required in a young patient, her ovaries can be left intact and she will retain her own hormonal levels. Radiation therapy avoids the risks of surgery and anesthesia, and offers a good chance of cure for more advanced stages of disease, and a low risk of complications. Since the ovaries are usually within the radiated field, castration or cessation of ovarian function occurs.

There does not appear to be any advantage to extending our surgery, or making it more radical. Current radiotherapy dosages and equipment are unlikely to be significantly improved in the coming decades.

There exists no curative chemotherapy for carcinoma of the cervix, and agents used for palliation usually achieve brief responses and are toxic. The possibility of the development of effective chemotherapy in the coming decades exists, although development of a single agent may take many years, and currently none of the experimental drugs being studied show promise. Lacking an effective agent, it is also not likely that adjunctive therapy, that is the addition of chemotherapy, will improve survival in patients treated with either surgery or radiation.

CARCINOMA OF THE ENDOMETRIUM

Carcinoma of the endometrium, a cancer of the lining of the uterus, appears to be more common in women who are obese, hypertensive, and have had few or no children. Exogenous estrogen therapy seems to be associated with a variant of endometrial carcinoma, and women who have hormonal imbalances which give them high levels of endogenous estrogen may also be at risk for developing this malignancy.

Fortunately, this disease becomes symptomatic early in its history, and is heralded by abnormal uterine bleeding or post-menopausal bleeding in a woman who has gone through cessation of her menstrual periods. Diagnosis is accomplished by biopsying the endometrium in an outpatient setting, or by performing a dilation and curettage of the uterus.

Prevention of this disease is tied to the removal of obesity as a risk factor, and correction of any underlying endocrinopathies in women in the reproductive years. However, since this disease is most common in the menopausal years, demonstrating that you are able to prevent cancer would require intervention plus followup for several decades. Again, our understanding of the disease allows us to screen populations at risk and to advise aggressive followup of abnormal or postmenopausal bleeding, but in a given case is only of value in assisting us to recognize a specific patient at risk, and not in preventing the disease. Further, recognition of abnormal or postmenopausal bleeding as the key symptom of this disease only allows early diagnosis of the cancer, which means we will be detecting the disease in earlier stages where it is more curable, but not preventing the disease.

Recognition of the occurrence of endometrial carcinoma in women who are placed on long term estrogen therapy for menopausal symptoms initially led many physicians and the public to decry estrogen replacement therapy, and argue for its elimination. However, recognition of the morbidity and mortality of osteoporosis, which results from loss of endogenous estrogens, and development of safe regimens of administration (relying heavily on progestational agents to oppose the estrogens), has led to a more reasonable philosophy wherein estrogen replacement therapy is safely administered in a cyclic fashion under close physician supervision. While not entirely eliminating risks, this should prevent the development of overt malignancies, and provide protection from the devastating consequences of osteoporosis, as well as relieving vaginal dryness, "hot flashes," and urinary discomfort secondary to tissue atrophy.

Current treatment of diagnosed endometrial carcinoma relies on combining a nonradical hysterectomy (removal only of the uterus and of the tubes and ovaries), and then, in selected patients, the addition of radiation therapy. Cure rates of early stage disease, which is what most patients fortunately present with, is quite acceptable and morbidity from treatment is low. Again, improvements in radiation or surgical techniques are unlikely. Future developments will probably rely on selecting out those patients who may not need both treatment modalities and can be spared unnecessary treatment and expense. Also, the future will likely see us developing means of pathologically studying hysterectomy specimens and thereby predicting patients with a high likelihood of recurrent cancer. These patients can then be treated with adjuvant chemotherapy, that is, chemotherapy added to surgery and/or radiation. Currently anti-estrogen hormones, or progestational agents, have an approximately 30% response rate in this disease with little or no associated toxicity. Analogs of these drugs are likely to be developed, and there is a real possibility of effective chemotherapy for this disease being developed in coming years.

OVARIAN CARCINOMA

While carcinoma of the endometrium and carcinoma of the cervix are more common, ovarian carcinoma is responsible for more fatalities. Ovarian carcinoma is an insidious disease, which is discovered late in its natural history, with a low cure rate. As in other cancers of the reproductive tract, etiology is unknown, and in fact risk factors are poorly understood or defined.

The ovary is an intraperitoneal organ, on a mobile stalk, and can enlarge to many times its normal size without being readily apparent. In addition, it is in free contact with the rest of the peritoneal cavity and metastasis or spread to intraabdominal organs, such as the large and small bowel, under surface of the diaphragm, and throughout the pelvis, are common.

Considerable research has been expended attempting to identify a serum marker, which would allow mass screening and early diagnosis of ovarian carcinoma. There have been exciting developments within the last few years, which hold promise; and very preliminary trials using these serum markers to screen populations at risk and patients with known disease are underway. Until such a screening serum test is available, the only method of screening large numbers of asymptomatic females is the annual physical exam, including a thorough rectovaginal examination. However, it is estimated that 10,000 examinations of asymptomatic women must be performed to find one patient with early stage ovarian carcinoma.

Current management of a pelvic mass is based on an awareness of the lethality and danger of missing ovarian carcinoma. Therefore, a prompt evaluation, and, if necessary, surgical exploration is warranted when an adnexal mass is found, and benign disease cannot be definitively proven. Delay in properly evaluating and diagnosing ovarian carcinoma can profoundly affect a patient's chance for cure.

When found, proper therapy for ovarian carcinoma is surgical removal of all visible tumor, followed by aggressive multi-agent chemotherapy. Only a few years ago, the best survival which could be anticipated was in the neighborhood of 30% at two years. However, proper surgical treatment combined with aggressive multi-agent chemotherapy now gives us a two year survival of over 70%, and in some instances, even those not cured may be anticipated to survive four or more years, leading a good quality life.

Modern chemotherapy involves close surveillance of the patient, and this careful monitoring prevents or minimizes toxicity to normal tissues. Many of the regimens can be administered on an outpatient basis, and patients are able to work or care for their families while undergoing treatment. Considerable research is underway to find analogs of current chemotherapeutic agents which have less toxicity, and at the same time increasing efforts are being made to develop means of controlling nausea and vomiting and other chemotherapeutic side effects.

Scanning of the abdomen and pelvis with ultrasound, computerized axial tomography (CAT) scans, and now nuclear magnetic resonance imaging have all been proposed as improvements in diagnosis and managing. However, clinical studies thus far have not confirmed the value of these newer dynamic imaging techniques, and thorough physical exam and close physician monitoring remain the keys to management and diagnosis of ovarian carcinoma.

VULVAR AND VAGINAL MALIGNANCIES

Cancer of the vagina and vulva are rare, and limited almost exclusively to the very elderly. Management is based on radical surgery or radiation, and improved quality of support services, i.e., anesthesia and blood banking, have made the operations safe, complications few, and survival good.

Controversy exists over whether cancer of the vulva and vagina have preinvasive lesions which develop into the cancer. However, when epithelial abnormalities are detected in the vagina or vulva, standard management is destruction of these lesions to remove any possibility of malignant progression, no matter how remote or theoretical. While in the past this required surgery with attendant scarring, the acceptance and use of laser surgery now provides a cosmetically acceptable means of destroying these lesions without causing disfigurement. In the future one may anticipate more extensive use of laser surgery, as well as more innovative use of the instrument to replace conventional surgery. The results should be surgery which causes less blood loss, less destruction of normal tissues, and better cosmetic result, without diminishing chances for cure.

GENERAL INNOVATIVE THERAPEUTICS

In addition to defining specific surgical, radiotherapeutic and/or chemotherapeutic treatment modalities for all of the gynecologic malignancies, recently we have seen the development of general medical interventions which allow cancer patients to undergo treatments considered too debilitating in the past. For example, total parenteral nutrition (TPN) now allows complete nutritional support to be given to a patient who is either cachectic from her underlying malignancy, or who as a result of treatment is unable to absorb sufficient calories to maintain bodily integrity. The ability to provide complete nutritional requirements by vein, not only allows us to overcome nutritional deficits caused by cancer or cancer related treatment, but also allows attempts at more aggressive resection of the abdominal organs. It is even now possible to provide total parenteral nutrition by vein while the patient is at home, and several commercial services are available which will monitor the patient and assist her and her family in maintaining safe parenteral nutrition. These patients can then go about their activities at home, and, to a limited extent, return to normal activities. Anticipated improvements in this technique may ultimately lead to the rare use of TPN in a hospital setting.

The devastating infections that were previously associated with cancer surgery are now uncommon due to developments of better antibiotics, to an appreciation of the multi-bacterial infections that were encountered, to a better understanding of the bacteria involved, and to improvement in surgical technique on the bowel which minimizes contamination and infection. These newer antibiotics combined with careful monitoring have reduced infections during intensive chemotherapy and are nearly always resolvable.

Reconstructive surgery, particularly creation of a neo-vagina, has led to restoration of sexual function in patients who have undergone extensive pelvic surgery. The increasing use of skin grafts and myocutaneous grafts, as well as omental slings, has in many cases allowed satisfactory reconstruction of a vagina permitting normal intercourse.

Use of automatic staplers to perform bowel anastomoses, as well as a better understanding of the blood supply to the bowel, the necessity of a bowel prep, and the limitations of radiation fields, have allowed bowel resections and reanastomoses to occur more safely, often saving the patient from permanent stoma. One could anticipate further improvements in this field, and hopefully an even more infrequent need for permanent diversion of the bowel or urinary tract.

Along with technical innovations and better support services, has come a marked improvement in patient education and consumerism. Recognition that cancer is not one disease, but rather hundreds of different diseases, must increase. Along with this the public must become more aware that cure, and prolonged survival, are already possible and the situation is getting better. The role of environmental carcinogens in malignancy of the reproductive tract remains problematic and warrants extensive further study. How this will be accomplished at a time when funding for basic research is diminishing is unclear, but one can only hope increasing consumer interest in medical care and basic science will lead to greater government and third party support for research on the etiology of genital cancer.

Increasing patient awareness has now led to an understanding of the need for second opinions. Further public awareness should lead to less reliance on quack remedies and more appropriate use of the latest information available to the medical and lay professions. Most patients with cancer continue to be treated by non-cancer specialists, in non-cancer centers. The government is funding programs aimed at bringing the latest developments in cancer research and treatment to community hospitals, and cancer centers are developing increasingly sophisticated computer systems for relaying information to out-lying physicians. The rapidity of modern communication systems should allow almost instant dissemination of the latest diagnostic and treatment modalities, and should allow in the foreseeable future a single level of excellent cancer care to be universally available.

REFERENCES

Henderson, C.I., & Conellos, G.P. (1980). Cancer of the breast: The past decade. *New England Journal of Medicine, 302,* 17-30.

Morrow, C.P., & Townsend, D.E. (1981). *Synopsis of gynecologic oncology.* New York: Wiley and Sons.

Moskowitz, M. (1983). Screening for breast cancer: How effective are our tests? *Ca-A Cancer Journal for Clinicians, 33,* 26-39.

Sontag, S. (1978). *Illness as metaphor.* New York: Ferrar, Strauss and Giroux.

Silverberg, E., & Lubera, J.A. (1983). A review of American Cancer Society estimates of cancer cases and deaths. *Ca-A Cancer Journal for Clinicians, 33,* 2-25.

Hypertension in Women:
Progress and Unsolved Problems

Lawrence R. Krakoff, MD

ABSTRACT. Hypertension is the most common cause of increased risk for heart and vascular disease in the adult population. Both men and women are at risk for hypertension and both benefit from anti-hypertensive therapy. However, hypertension tends to be less prevalent in women and is better tolerated; hypertensive women have fewer strokes and heart attacks than do hypertensive men. Women may develop reversible hypertension due to use of birth control pills. Another form of curable secondary hypertension, renal artery stenosis caused by fibromuscular dysplasia, is much more frequent in young women than men. Antihypertensive drug treatment for severe hypertension benefits both sexes, although clinical trials establishing this have been conducted only in men. There is no proof that white women with mild hypertension benefit from antihypertensive drug therapy. Non-drug approaches including weight reduction, change in diet, and exercise may be equally beneficial.

INTRODUCTION

Hypertension or high blood pressure is the most common disorder of the cardiovascular system in adults. Simply put, hypertension is an elevation of pressure in the systemic arteries, those bearing blood from the heart to all tissues outside of the chest. In part, hypertension is defined by statistical techniques defining that segment of the population at the upper 10-15% of the distribution of arterial pressure for each age (Epstein, 1982). Another, more important basis for defining high arterial pressure is the level at which an increase in cardiovascular disease occurs. On this basis, as many as 50% of some populations may be considered to have hypertension (Kannel, 1983).

Elevated arterial pressure and its risk for a higher percentage of future cardiovascular disease occurs in both men and women. There is reason to believe that both sexes benefit from reduction of arterial pressure in the prevention of future cardiovascular morbidity.

Despite these similarities, there are distinct differences between men and women with regard to some of the patterns of high blood pressure, the relationship between high blood pressure and cardiovascular morbidity, causes of hypertension, and the expected benefit to be gained by reduction of arterial pressure through the use of antihypertensive drugs. This review will focus upon the most clearcut differences between men and women with regard to hypertension. It will also emphasize several specific areas where there is need for additional research that should lead to better medical management for those women who have high blood pressure and may be thus at risk for future cardiovascular disease.

EPIDEMIOLOGIC CONSIDERATIONS

Among the various factors that might be related to having high blood pressure, several have been well studied, including family history, racial background, and sex. High blood pressure tends to cluster in families implying a very strong genetic component in its etiology. In the United States, blacks tend to have more hypertension than whites. Overall, men tend to be slightly more hypertensive than women when matched for age and race. An example from the High Blood Pressure Detection and Followup Study (1977) is shown in Table 1.

The impact of hypertension, that is the development of cardiovascular disease among those who are hypertensive, is quite different between men and women. In several long-term follow-up studies, it has been demonstrated that women "tolerate" hypertension better than men by having fewer strokes and far fewer heart attacks (Kannel, 1983). When race and sex are considered, it is apparent that black men have the highest cardiovascular morbidity due to hyper-

Table 1. Prevalence of Hypertension in the First Screen of the High Blood Pressure Detection and Follow-up Study (HDFP)

White		Black	
Men	Women	Men	Women
13.5%	8.4%	28.1%	23.1%

Hypertension was defined by a seated diastolic blood pressure of 95 mm Hg or more taken in the home by a trained observer.

tension, black women and white men have nearly similar rates of cardiovascular disease when hypertensive, and white women experience the lease cardiovascular morbidity due to high blood pressure. Despite the large number of studies on hypertension that have been performed in recent years, these differences remain unexplained.

CAUSES OF HYPERTENSION

More than 90% of those who have hypertension have no detectable cause for this disorder when tested by usual medical diagnostic techniques. The term "essential hypertension" is applied to these patients. However, this term indicates only that the cause of the condition remains unknown. In recent years, there have been attempts to subdivide "essential" hypertension into different subgroups which may lead to the detection of underlying causative mechanisms. Best known for subgrouping of the essential hypertensive population is the technique of renin-profiling. The renin-angiotensin system is a complex protein-peptide hormone system which is controlled by the release of the enzyme, renin, from the kidney. This occurs in response to alterations in arterial pressure, salt balance and the effect of norepinephrine and epinephrine, catecholamines released by the sympathetic nervous system (Brunner & Gavras, 1982).

Briefly, essential hypertensives may be considered low, normal, or high renin subtypes. Evidence suggests that the low renin subgroups are more likely to have high blood pressure because of salt and water retention when compared with their normal or high renin counterparts (Gavras & Brunner, 1982). In contrast, some of the high renin patients show patterns suggesting an abnormal overactivity of the sympathetic nervous system causing renin release through the activation of renal beta adrenergic receptors. In general, high renin essential hypertensives tend to be younger, white, and equally male or female. In contrast, low renin hypertensives tend to be older, black, and female. These broad generalizations obscure the fact that there are many exceptions and that there is need for much additional research in defining the various subgroups of essential hypertension and the mechanisms that account for high blood pressure.

There are several well-defined causes of high blood pressure resulting from derangements in kidney function or in oversecretion by the endocrine glands. High blood pressure due to a defined disturbance of this type is referred to as secondary hypertension. These are indicated in Table 2. High blood pressure due to narrowing of the renal arteries (renal artery stenosis) is most often a result of atherosclerotic occlusion of one or both main renal arteries. The predisposing factors to atherosclerosis including hypertension itself, elevated serum lipids, smoking, or diabetes are the major factors which account for atherosclerotic renal artery narrowing. In contrast, a less common form of renal artery stenosis is due to the fibromuscular dysplasias—a group of disorders of the renal artery wall which appear to be a result of abnormal growth patterns of one or more layers of this artery. Renal artery stenosis due to fibromuscular dysplasia is far more common in women than men and appears in adolescence or early adulthood (Kaplan, 1978). Other causes of secondary hypertension tend to occur with almost equal frequency in women and men.

One form of secondary hypertension that only occurs in women is that due to the use of oral contraceptive pills (Krakoff, 1982). Oral contraceptive hypertension was described shortly after the use of birth control pills became widespread. While overt hypertension due to oral contraceptive use occurred in a very small fraction of those women who used this form of contraception, population studies suggested that a small increase in arterial pressure occurred in a large number of women who employed this form of birth control. The long-term effect of small upward changes of arterial pressure within the normotensive range remains to be established.

Table 2. Causes of Secondary Hypertension

```
Disorders of the Kidneys
      Renal artery stenosis
            Atherosclerosis
            Fibromuscular dysplasia
      Chronic renal diseases
      Obstruction of the urinary outflow tracts

Disorders of the Adrenal Cortex
      Primary aldosteronism
      Cushing's syndrome - hypercortisolism

Pheochromocytoma - catecholamine-producing tumor

Coarctation of the Aorta

Oral Contraceptive Hypertension
```

Women who use oral contraceptive pills have a greater tendency to stroke at an early age compared to normal women not using the pill. This effect appears due to the clotting action of oral contraceptives, rather than the effect of the pill on blood pressure. It has been suggested that women who use the oral contraceptive pill and also smoke have a higher likelihood of premature coronary artery disease. Again, this appears to be due to effects of the oral contraceptive components upon factors in addition to arterial pressure, per se.

TREATMENT OF HYPERTENSION: DIFFERENCES BETWEEN MEN AND WOMEN

There is no doubt that the use of anti-hypertensive drugs has had a major impact in reducing the likelihood of cardiovascular disease. This was first shown in well-controlled randomized clinical trials conducted by the Veterans Administration Cooperative Study Group on Antihypertensive Agents (1970). As might be expected, only men were enrolled for these studies. Nonetheless, these formed the basis for the initial view that severe hypertension should invariably be treated with anti-hypertensive drugs to achieve normalization of arterial pressure. Subsequent clinical trials have been conducted to assess the effect of anti-hypertensive drug therapy in milder forms of hypertension, defined as pretreatment diastolic pressures in the range of 90-105 mm Hg. Most of these have demonstrated benefit of anti-hypertensive therapy through reduction of stroke with little obvious effect upon coronary heart disease (Krakoff, 1983).

All but one of the recent clinical trials devoted to assessing the effect of anti-hypertensive therapy have been conducted on men. In contrast, the trial conducted by the High Blood Pressure Detection and Follow-up Program Cooperative Group (1979) included men and women, blacks and whites. Some of the results of this study are given in Table 3. It is important to recognize that the design of the HDFP study departed somewhat from the traditional clinical trial. After screening a large population in order to select those at risk because of hypertension, patients were divided into two groups for management. One group was given anti-hypertensive medication in specially designed clinics employing strict protocols, intensive follow-up, and re-evaluation. This special care group was compared to those randomly selected for return to clinical care in their com-

Table 3. All Cause Mortality in the HDFP Study by Sex and Race
after 5 Years of Treatment

	Special Care Clinics	Referred Case (Community)	% Reduction for Special Care
Black men	10.6	13.0	18.5
Black women	5.2	7.2	27.8
White men	5.8	6.8	14.7
White women	4.9	4.8	-2.1

Rates are expressed per 100 patients.

munities by whatever mechanism was available. There was then no untreated group or placebo control as is usually the case in therapeutic trials. Because of the design of the HDFP trial, it is extremely difficult to determine which factors specifically caused the outcome. Nonetheless, it is apparent that among those managed in the special care clinics, when compared with their counterparts, there is evidence of benefit in black men, black women, white men, but not white women. Perhaps these differences are due to the epidemiologic trends for untreated disease that were mentioned before. Another possibility is that white women tend to seek medical care with greater frequency than the other subgroups and thus benefited equally from the resources available to them in their communities. Nonetheless, at the present time there is less evidence that anti-hypertensive therapy is beneficial for white women, a group which has the greatest longevity in the American population. There is also no evidence that anti-hypertensive drug therapy is harmful for women, although the question has not been addressed in the same way as it has in men.

The recently published Multiple Risk Factor Intervention Trial (1982) conducted only in men at risk for coronary heart disease, raises several pertinent questions. This trial compared men in the upper 25% for risk of future coronary heart disease because of smoking, elevated cholesterol, or high blood pressure treated in special care centers or referred to their community resources. Anti-hypertensive therapy per se had no statistically significant benefit. However, in subgroups selected for pre-existing electrocardiographic abnormalities, those enrolled in the special care clinics did *worse* because of the higher occurrence of deaths due to cardiovascular disease. It has been suggested, but not yet proven, that the excessive use of diuretic drugs causing potassium loss in the special care clinics might account for this difference. Nonetheless, this study raises the issue of whether or not some forms of anti-hypertensive drug therapy might be harmful and focuses attention on nonpharmacologic methods for reduction of arterial pressure especially in those with mild forms of hypertension.

The foregoing discussion indicates that the use of anti-hypertensive drugs should be re-evaluated especially for those who are least likely to benefit from them, i.e., white women. While few would suggest that blood pressure reduction is not beneficial, the means for blood pressure reduction must now be scrutinized for maximum safety. Among older hypertensive women, there is some evidence that sensitivity to salt may be a significant issue. On this basis, reduction of dietary salt might be useful. However, recent evidence suggests that other dietary constituents might provide a basis for alternate therapy. A highly controversial recently published article suggests that mild elevations of arterial pressure in the population at large might be linked to dificiencies in dietary calcium and potassium (McCarron, Morris, Henry, & Stanton, 1984). This is of special interest for older women in whom osteoporosis poses such a threat. The question can be asked whether supplemental dietary calcium might not be doubly beneficial in prevention of osteoporosis and reduction of arterial pressure. Clearly, appropriate research is necessary to address this problem and arrive at a well-documented recommendation for those at risk.

Anti-hypertensive drugs have been in a continuing state of development since the initial application of diuretics and of reserpine for blood pressure reduction. There are now more than 30 separate individual anti-hypertensive drugs available for use in the United States plus the various combination forms that have been marketed. There is no perfect anti-hypertensive medication. Side effects or adverse reactions of some form have occurred with each. Among those adverse reactions more pertinent to women are the effects of several centrally acting anti-hypertensive anti-adrenergic drugs (those that act within the brain to reduce the activity of the sympathetic nervous system). Two of these, methyldopa and reserpine, cause increased secretion of prolactin by the pituitary gland which may lead to galactorrhea i.e., inappropriate formation and secretion of breast milk (Turkington, 1972).

It was once reported that use of reserpine, one of the oldest anti-hypertensive drugs, might be associated with the development of breast cancer, but subsequent epidemiologic research failed to confirm this association (Mack et al., 1975). Another anti-hypertensive diuretic, spirolactone, has a progesterone-like action and may cause menstrual irregularities in women. Surprisingly, this same drug causes breast growth (gynecomastia) in men which may become quite painful. Impotence is a reported adverse reaction of many antihypertensive drugs given to men. Several of the anti-andrenergic drugs that interfere with sympathetic nervous function impair normal ejaculation. The effect of the various anti-hypertensive drugs upon sexual function in women has not been well described. There is also a lack of detailed descriptions of the effects of these agents upon the various hormone systems that are unrelated to cardiovascular control.

CONCLUSIONS

National statistics indicate a reduction in the frequency of cerebrovascular accidents and in coronary heart disease (Stamler & Liu, 1983). Such findings imply that prevention of cardiovascular disease through the treatment of high blood pressure has been successful. Maximizing this success, however, means recognizing the difference between subgroups of those at greater and lesser risk because of hypertension and of proceeding with the necessary research for defining the most appropriate, beneficial, and least harmful form of blood pressure reduction. For women with mild hypertension, there are many problems to solve before ideal anti-hypertensive management can be attained. There is little doubt, however, that women with more severe hypertension benefit greatly from the knowledge that has been achieved through clinical trials that enrolled men only.

REFERENCES

Brunner, H.R., & Gavras, H. (1982). Renin angiotensin, aldosterone, salt, and the kidney. In H.R. Brunner & H. Gavras (Eds.). Clinical hypertension and hypotension (pp. 209-228). New York and Basel: Marcel Dekker, Inc.

Epstein, F.S. (1982). The problem of hypertension. In H.R. Brunner & H. Gavras (Eds.). Clinical hypertension and hypotension (pp. 3-21). New York and Basel: Marcel Dekker, Inc.

Gavras, H., & Brunner, H.R. (1982). Essential hypertension. In H.R. Brunner & H. Gavras (Eds.). Clinical hypertension and hypotension (pp. 165-177). New York and Basel: Marcel Dekker, Inc.

Hypertension Detection and Follow-Up Program Cooperative Group. (1977). The Hypertension Detection and Follow-Up Program: A progress report. *Circulation Research, 40*(5) (supp. I), I-106-I-109.

Hypertension Detection and Follow-Up Program Cooperative Group. (1979). Five-year findings of the Hypertension Detection and Follow-up Program. II. Mortality by race-sex and age. *Journal of the American Medical Association, 242*(23), 2572-2577.

Kannel, W.B. (1983). An overview of the risk factors for cardiovascular disease. In N.M. Kaplan & J. Stamler (Eds.), *Prevention of coronary heart disease: Practical management of the risk factors* (pp. 1-19). Philadelphia: WB Saunders.

Kaplan, N.M. (1978). Renovascular hypertension and renin-secreting tumors. In *Clinical hypertension,* 2nd ed. (Chapter 7, pp. 218-260). Baltimore: Williams & Wilkins.

Krakoff, L.R. (1982). Oral contraceptive hypertension. In H.R. Brunner & H. Gavras (Eds.), *Clinical hypertension and hypotension* (pp. 137-150). New York and Basel: Marcel Dekker, Inc.

Krakoff, L. (1983). Changing strategies in the management of hypertension. *Cardiovascular Reviews & Reports, 4*(3), 319-324.

Mack, T.M., Henderson, B.E., Gerkins, V.R., Arthur, M., Baptista, J., & Pike, M.C. (1975). Reserpine and breast cancer in a retirement community. *New England Journal of Medicine, 292*(26), 1366-1371.

McCarron, D.A., Morris, C.D., Henry, H.J., & Stanton, J.L. (1984). Blood pressure and nutrient intake in the United States. *Science, 224,* 1392-1398.

Multiple Risk Factor Intervention Trial Research Group. (1982). Multiple Risk Factor Intervention Trial: Risk factor changes and mortality results. *Journal of the American Medical Association, 248*(12), 1465-1477.

Stamler, J., & Liu, K. (1983). The benefits of prevention. In N.M. Kaplan & J. Stamler (Eds.), *Prevention of coronary heart disease: Practical management of the risk factors* (pp. 188-207). Philadelphia: WB Saunders.

Turkington, R.W. (1972). Prolactin secretion in patients treated with various drugs. *Archives of Internal Medicine, 130,* 349-357.

Veterans Administration Cooperative Study Group on Antihypertensive Agents. (1970). Effects of treatment on morbidity in hypertension. II. Results in patients with diastolic blood pressure averaging 90 through 114 mm Hg. *Journal of the American Medical Association, 213*(7), 1143-1152.

Common Eye Problems
in the Older Woman

Ann M. Bajart, MD

ABSTRACT. Dry eye syndrome, cataracts, glaucoma, and macular degeneration are the four most common eye problems affecting elderly women. The cause, symptomatology, treatment, and prognosis of each condition are discussed.

The elderly woman is subject to many common eye problems such as dry eyes and cataracts simply by virtue of having survived to the time when these problems are a normal and natural occurrence. Degenerative conditions such as macular degeneration and chronic diseases such as glaucoma cause slow, progressive ocular changes with cumulative loss of vision and often occur in the seventh and eighth decades of life concomitantly with cataracts.

DRY EYES

Drying of the ocular surface is a major cause of symptoms in the adult population. The usual complaint is one of eye fatigue and heaviness after reading for more than ten or fifteen minutes. Vision becomes blurred and the eyes begin to feel hot and tired. There is often the desire to close and rest the eyes. Headache is not a problem. In more severe cases there may be constant foreign body sensation as if there were dust or an eyelash in the eye. Some patients complain about difficulty opening their eyes in the morning as if the eyes were sewn shut, as opposed to being crusted shut as with a lid infection. Frequently there will be a ropey mucus present at the nasal corner of the lids that is very rubbery when wiped away. Paradoxically, tearing may be the presenting symptom of dryness. Symptoms are usually worse in dry environments, in the wind, and with exposure to irritating fumes from cleaning products or smoke.

The cause of ocular dryness is decreased basal tear secretion from the lacrimal and accessory lacrimal glands (Weil, 1983). In children tear secretion is plentiful. About the age of twenty, however, there is a definite reduction of reflex tearing which continues to decrease over time (Jones, 1966). Birth control pills, diuretics, anti-histamines, anti-depressants, and anti-cholinergic medications further diminish tear secretion. Rheumatoid arthritis is frequently accompanied by ocular dryness. Decreased or incomplete reflex blinking aggravates dryness because the tear film rests along the lower lid margin. If the upper lid does not fully close with a blink, the tear film will not be spread evenly across the front surface of the eye by the squeegee action of the upper lid; then the cornea and conjunctiva will become dry and chapped. Similar problems occur if the lower lids are irregular in contour or in abnormal contact with the globe (Silver, 1983). It is the chapping of the surface that causes the symptoms. When the surface is badly chapped the simple movement of the upper lid across the irritated surface causes more irritation and a vicious cycle of non-blinking, increased dryness, increased irritation, decreased or less complete blinking begins. At this point the eyes may become so irritated that reflex tearing is stimulated and the patient presents with a chief complaint of excess tearing!

The diagnosis of a dry eye can be made by examining the eyes using a slit-lamp microscope and instilling flouroscein or rose Bengal stain. The eyes are usually quite white and quiet looking on direct examination with a flashlight. With the stain, the dry irritated cells pick up the yellow or red color in a very fine punctate fashion in the area between the lids. The staining is usually most pronounced in the lower third of the exposed cornea and conjunctiva appearing as if they had been blasted with very fine sand. The conjunctiva in the area of the lower lateral lid margin is frequently clear but mildly swollen and jelly-like. The baseline tear secretion is tested by instilling anesthetic eye drops and small calibrated strips of filter paper over the lower lids into the lower tear lake. The strips act like wicks absorbing the tears secreted over a five minute period. The results are reported as millimeters of wetting of the strip. A severely dry eye may show zero wetting as opposed to fifteen millimeters for a normal eye. The test is referred to as a Schirmer test.

Treatment consists of keeping the eyes lubricated. In mild cases all that may be necessary is to make the patient aware of the fact that her blink is incomplete or infrequent and that she should concentrate on blinking fully and more frequently as soon as she is aware of her eyes. This is especially common among contact lens wearers or in patients who become symptomatic after extended close work or reading.

Artificial tears are the mainstay of treatment for the dry eye. There are approximately twenty different brands available without prescription. Patients tend to develop a brand preference just as they have a preference for shampoo or toothpaste so they should be encouraged to try different brands if they find one type unsatisfactory. Complaints that the artificial tears hurt and burn when instilled are an indication for more frequent instillation of the tears or the addition of an ointment rather than an indication for cessation of treatment. Just as plain water is painful to severely chapped skin, tears are initially painful to severely dry eyes. Patients may be instructed to use the drops up to every hour depending upon the degree of their symptoms. If they are still symptomatic they should use bland lubricant ointment such as Lacri-Lube, Duolube or Duratears up to every three hours while awake and at bedtime. The ointment prevents evaporation of whatever tears the patient can produce but also causes a greasy blur of vision. Some patients manage by staggering the time of instillation between the two eyes.

Humidification of the patient's living and working environments is a necessary adjunct of therapy. This usually requires the use of room sized humidifiers during the heating season although a small humidifier is better than none at all. Avoidance of wind, dust, smoke, and known irritants may not be possible but should be minimized; sunglasses are often useful as windshields. The patient should become aware of her environment and potential environments and should be encouraged to anticipate situations which will aggravate dryness and which will require more lubrication than usual such as air-conditioned rooms and automobiles, airplanes, deserts. It is important for the patient to respond to minimal symptoms because treatment is much more difficult and time consuming when the eye becomes severely symptomatic.

The prognosis for the dry eye patient is good once the patient learns to use lubricants on a frequent basis and to avoid aggravating factors. There is no cure for the dry eye but it is rarely disabling or blinding.

CATARACT

Cataracts are an inevitable consequence of aging. They are the commonest cause of painless progressive visual loss in the elderly. A cataract is an optical opacification of the normally transparent lens of the eye. There are many specific types of cataracts. They may be due to aging, drugs, environmental, or metabolic factors and it is common to have more than one type. People generally develop symptomatic nuclear cataracts which are related to aging after the seventh decade of life. The lens of the human eye begins to form during the sixth week of gestation. It continues to grow throughout life laying down concentric layers of lens material in analogous fashion to the growth of a deciduous tree trunk. The central lens consists of the oldest lens fibers which were formed during the embryonic period while the outer layer consists of the newest. Over time the lens becomes physically thicker and less flexible. By the mid-forties the internal muscles of the eye have difficulty maintaining flexion of the lens so that the eye can focus for close vision. This is the reason most adults begin to need reading glasses in their forties. As the aging process continues the central lens fibers lose their nuclei and become more condensed (Cotlier, 1981). The central lens or nucleus develops a light amber yellow pigmentation which will slowly increase over many years sometimes becoming cola brown. This is called a nuclear cataract. Its effect upon vision is to filter out light like an internal sunglass. Consequently individuals with nuclear cataracts require stronger light to see. Because the increased density of the nucleus changes the refractive index of the lens, they also become more nearsighted and have more trouble seeing at distance than reading.

Posterior subcapsular cataracts develop on the back layer of the lens. They may occur in younger individuals but usually after the fifth decade. They are sometimes caused by prolonged use of steroids for systemic diseases such as asthma, colitis, arthritis, or inflammatory skin conditions. The cataract appears as a frosting of the posterior lens capsule and is best seen with the ophthalmoscope and a dilated pupil against a red reflex. Patients with a posterior subcapsular cataract complain about markedly decreased vision in direct light and will have more difficulty with reading than with distance vision. Vision may be quite good when tested in a dark room where the pupils are relatively large but decreases significantly when the room is made bright and the pupils constrict.

At the present time the only treatment for cataracts is surgical removal. There are no laser medical treatments available. However, the presence of a cataract is NOT an indication for its removal. Cataract extraction is indicated if the cataract is interfering with the patient's ability to function visually at a level needed for a happy productive daily life. Visual needs must be determined for each individual.

Cataract surgery is highly successful (in the range of 95%) but there is always the possibility of severe complication such as hemorrhage or infection that may even result in loss of the eye. For this reason surgery should be done only when the cataract is causing visual dysfunction.

Removal of the cataract will not restore vision. After the natural lens of the eye is removed the eye cannot clearly focus light. It is necessary to correct the vision with glasses, with a contact lens, or with a lens implanted inside the eye at the time of surgery. Glasses were the most common method of correction of aphakia (absence of the lens) prior to the last decade when intra-ocular lenses became better developed and more widely employed. Patients, especially the elderly, have a very difficult time adjusting to cataract glasses which cause a 25-30% disparity between the normal and aphakic image size; they also have to relearn depth perception and adjust to a constricted visual field. In addition, the patient cannot see out of both eyes with cataract glasses unless both eyes are aphakic because the brain cannot fuse a normal size and a magnified image. Contact lenses eliminate the problems of restricted field and decrease magnification to 7% but some elderly patients cannot tolerate contacts for physical or psychological reasons (Milder & Rubin, 1978). Even with an implanted intra-ocular lens spectacles are required for best corrected distance or reading vision or both.

GLAUCOMA

Glaucoma is a disease causing visual loss due to elevated intra-ocular pressure. It affects approximately 2% of the population over the age of forty. Its morbidity can be prevented or minimized by proper diagnosis and treatment. It is usually asymptomatic until there has been severe, irreversible visual loss. For this reason it is important to screen patients over forty on a routine basis every two to three years for elevated intra-ocular pressure. It is especially important if there is a positive family history of glaucoma since it is a hereditary disease. Intra-ocular pressure is completely different from systemic blood pressure and must be measured specifically.

The pressure inside the eye is determined by the rate of production of aqueous fluid by the ciliary body inside the eye and the rate of outflow of the fluid through the drainage channels that are located circumferentially in the front of the eye in the angle formed by the dome-shaped cornea and the iris. Since the eye is a closed system the pressure will rise if the inflow excedes the outflow. When the internal eye pressure rises it exerts pressure on the blood vessels within the eye and may strangulate them. The nerve tissue around the optic nerve is most sensitive to the effects of increased pressure because it cannot regenerate once it is severely damaged by decreased blood supply. As nerve fibers die, corresponding small areas of blindness develop. The first blind areas are in the peripheral nasal field of vision or surrounding but not involving the central vision. Since the nasal fields of the right and left eyes overlap, the patient is most often totally unaware of the visual loss.

The diagnosis of glaucoma is made by measuring the pressure, examining the drainage angle using a gonioscopy lens, examining the optic disc and plotting the visual field. The normal range of intraocular pressure is between 10 and 22 mm Hg. Glaucoma may occur in patients whose pressures are sometimes in the normal range. Eye pressure normally fluctuates 2-3mm Hg in a diurnal curve. In glaucoma the range of fluctuation can be markedly greater than normal (Chandler & Grant, 1979). Thus it is very important to examine the optic disc to evaluate the extent of cupping. A cupped disc is highly suspicious for glaucoma even if the pressure is normal. It is possible to have glaucoma without any visual loss if the disease has been diagnosed early in its course. This is the reason for routine screening.

Treatment for open angle glaucoma initially consists of drops. Polypharmacy is the rule as the disease progresses since the various types of medication have different mechanisms of action which are synergistic or at least additive. The first line of treatment consists of beta-blockers such as timolol maleate (Timoptic) and/or epinephrine derivatives (Eppy-N, Glaucon, Epitrate et al.). They do not constrict the pupil and cause little visual disturbance as opposed to the cholinergic drugs such as pilocarpine, Carbachol, or cholinesterase inhibitors such as echothiophate iodide which constrict the pupil and act by increasing the facility of aqueous outflow through the trabecular meshwork in the angle. Systemic carbonic anhydrase inhibitors (Diamox, Neptazane) are added if further pressure reduction is needed.

The beta-blockers can cause significant systemic problems in patients with asthma, congestive heart failure, or A-V heart block.

They can also precipitate confusion in the elderly (Van Buskirk, 1980). The cholinergic eye drops have relatively few systemic side effects. Echothiophate iodide (Phosphaline Iodide) which inhibits the breakdown of acetylcholine can cause diarrhea, abdominal cramps, and general fatigue. Toxic systemic symptoms may not appear for weeks or months after the start of the drug. Carbonic anhydrase inhibitors frequently cause side effects such as tingling of the extremities, nausea, depression, and decreased libido. They cause acidosis and can precipitate kidney stones in susceptible individuals (Havener, 1983).

When maximum tolerated medical therapy still fails to keep the intra-ocular pressure under control laser surgery may be employed (Lustgarten et al., 1984). Laser trabeculoplasty (LTP) utilizes the highly focused light energy of a laser beam to burn holes in the drainage meshwork and increase the facility with which the intraocular fluid flows out of the eye. It is performed on an out-patient basis with little discomfort and relatively low risk. If LTP fails to control the pressure, conventional filtering surgery can be employed to create a shunt from within the eye to the potential space under the surface conjunctival tissue. The eye is actually entered so infection, hemorrhage, and cataract formation become risks of the surgery. The shunt may heal and scar with time causing the operation to fail. Filtering operations are often associated with decreased acuity, principally from cataract formation (Lewis & Phelps, 1984).

MACULAR DEGENERATION

Macular degeneration is the leading cause of legal blindness in the United States for adults over 60 years of age. The specific cause is unknown (Strahlman, Fine, & Hillis, 1983). It involves the area of the retina and choroid that are concerned with reading or central vision as opposed to the remaining retina which gives rise to peripheral vision. Macular changes can occur slowly over many years, beginning as asymptomatic discrete round yellow spots of retinal pigment epithelial atrophy (drusen) that are visible only with an ophthalmoscope. With time they increase in number and can coalesce. As the overlying photoreceptors degenerate visual symptoms begin, usually with complaints of distortion of letters or loss of a part of a letter while reading. As the degeneration progresses the distortion becomes greater and is noticeable when the patient is looking at faces and objects in the environment. In its advanced stages only peripheral vision remains and the object of regard disappears as the patient tries to look directly at it; it does not cause total blindness. The atrophic or "dry" form of macular degeneration is untreatable. Low vision aids can be prescribed to magnify the images seen by the less acute para-macular retina.

There is also a neovascular form of macular degeneration where abnormal fine blood vessels begin to grow under the retina. The new vessels leak and may bleed leading to subretinal scar formation and a rapid more profound loss of central vision. Neovascular macular degeneration is responsible for 88% of visual loss in eyes with senile macular degeneration (Berkow, 1984). Bressler, Bressler and Fine (1982) reported that 70% of central neovascular membranes eventually progressed to cause legal blindness. The time course from first detection of abnormal vessels to legal blindness was 21 months. The risk of neovascular maculopathy involving the second eye from the time of visual loss in the first eye was 13% by 12 months, 22% by 24 months, and 29% by 36 months. Fortunately, neovascular macular degeneration in not invariably bilateral. In Berkow's study 39% of patients with a neovascular macular scar in one eye had only dry senile macular changes in the fellow eye.

Patients with drusen or "dry" macular degeneration should be monitored for the onset of visual distortion which may indicate the appearance of neovascularization. They should report such symptoms to their ophthalmologists who should obtain a fluorescein angiogram if the physical findings are suspicious. Argon laser photocoagulation is beneficial in the preservation of vision in eyes where the neovascular membrane is 200 microns or more from the central fovea. Unfortunately such a location is relatively uncommon (Berkow, 1984).

SUMMARY

The older woman is subject to dry eyes and to cataract formation which are both so common as to be considered a normal part of the aging process. By having routine eye exams every three years after the age of forty, the patient can discuss her problems concerning visual or ocular discomfort with her ophthalmologist. Very frequently a careful examination including evaluation of the need for or a change in glasses and an explanation of the cause of the symptoms will be sufficient to allay the underlying fears of blindness. She may be advised to use lubricants in the case of dry eyes or better light for reading in the case of incipient cataracts. More importantly, she can be checked for glaucoma and have the retina examined for signs of damage from diabetes or high blood pressure of which she may be unaware. If such a condition were detected or suspected, appropriate medical therapy could be instituted to prevent progression of the pathological process. There is evidence that intense ultraviolet light increases the likelihood of cataract formation and retinal degeneration. Hence, it would be reasonable to avoid intense sunlight and to use ultraviolet filtering glasses when outside during daylight hours. Unfortunately, there are no simple eye washes nor exercises to prevent eye disease. Early detection of the cause of visual or ocular discomfort remains the critical factor. Regular examinations are recommended every three years from age forty to sixty and then every one to two years thereafter.

REFERENCES

Berkow, J.W. (1984). Subretinal neovascularization in senile macular degeneration. *American Journal of Ophthalmology, 97,* 143-147.

Bressler, S.B., Bressler, N.M., & Fine, S.L. (1982). The natural course of choroidal neovascular membranes. *American Journal of Ophthalmology, 93,* 157-163.

Chandler, P.A., & Grant, W.M. (1979). *Glaucoma.* Philadelphia: Lea and Febiger.

Cotlier, E. (1981). The lens. In R.A. Moses, (Ed.), *Adler's physiology of the eye* (7th ed.) (pp. 277-303). St Louis: C.V. Mosby.

Havener, W.H. (1983). *Ocular pharmacology* (5th ed). St. Lewis: C.V. Mosby.

Jones, L.T. (1966). The lacrimal secretory system and its treatment. *American Journal of Ophthalmology, 62,* 47-60.

Lewis, R.A., & Phelps, C.D. (1984). Trabeculectomy v thermosclerostomy. *Archives of Ophthalmology, 102,* 533-536.

Lustgarten, J., Podos, S.M., Ritch, R., Fischer, R., Stetz, D., Zborowski, L., & Boas, R. (1984). Laser trabeculoplasty. *Archives of Ophthalmology, 102,* 517-519.

Milder, B., & Rubin, M.L. (1978). *The fine art of prescribing glasses.* Gainesville, Florida: Triad Scientific Publishers.

Silver, B. (1983). Involutional changes and the lacrimal system. In B. Milder (Ed.), *The lacrimal system* (pp. 165-175). Norwalk, CT: Appleton Century Crofts.

Strahlman, E.R., Fine, S.L., & Hillis, A. (1983). The second eye of patients with senile macular degeneration. *Archives of Ophthalmology, 101,* 1191-1193.

Van Buskirk, E.M. (1980). Adverse reactions from timolol administration. *Ophthalmology, 87,* 447-450.

Weil, B.A. (1983). The dry eye. In B. Milder (Ed.), *The lacrimal system* (pp. 117-124). Norwalk, CT: Appleton Century Crofts.

Osteoporosis

Frederick S. Kaplan, MD

ABSTRACT. Osteoporosis is the leading cause of disabling and often life-threatening fractures in elderly women. This paper discusses risk factors in osteoporosis such as heredity, race, age, sex, diet, and exercise, as well as disease related causes of bone loss. Early symptoms, clinical findings, and currently used diagnostic techniques are reviewed. And the management of osteoporosis—both treatment of symptomatic disease and its sequelae, and preventive measures designed to maintain skeletal mass and integrity—is described.

Osteoporosis is a condition of decreased mass per unit volume of normally mineralized bone. It is the most common skeletal disorder in the world, and is second only to arthritis as a leading cause of musculoskeletal morbidity in the elderly.

The first symptoms occur when bone mass is so compromised that the skeletal framework can no longer withstand the mechanical stresses of everyday living. The most prevalent complications are compression fractures of the vertebral bodies and fractures of the ribs, proximal femur (hip) and humerus, and distal radius, all occurring with minimal trauma.

Of the numerous conditions that can deplete the skeletal mass and cause osteoporosis, the most common is postmenopausal bone loss. Every women in the perimenopausal age group is at risk, and as many as 15 million American women have symptomatic disease. Postmenopausal osteoporosis is the leading cause of fractures in the elderly (Garraway, Stauffer, Kurland, & O'Fallon, 1979).

POSTMENOPAUSAL AND AGE-RELATED OSTEOPOROSIS

The average American woman lives 25 years after the menopause. Of the 40 million women in the United States who are 50 years of age or older, more than half are likely to have radiographically detectable evidence of abnormally decreased bone mass (osteopenia) in the spine, and in more than a third, major orthopedic problems related to osteoporosis occur eventually. More than 80% of the 2 million fractures sustained by women over age 50 and most of the approximately 200,000 hip fractures that occur in the United States each year are secondary to osteoporosis. The current cost for acute care of patients with osteoporotic injuries exceeds $3 billion annually (Kelsey, White, Pastides, & Bisbee, 1979).

Age-related osteoporosis occurs in both men and women, and is caused by bone loss that accompanies aging. Bone mass peaks after skeletal maturity some time in the third decade. The size of this bank stays nearly constant throughout much of adult life, with the body redistributing its assets according to structural needs. With age, the balance between bone formation and resorption rates is disturbed, leading to a decrease in bone mass (Ivey & Baylink, 1981).

RISK FACTORS IN OSTEOPOROSIS

The many factors that influence attainment and maintenance of peak bone mass also determine who is at risk of osteoporosis. The person most likely to be affected is a sedentary, postmenopausal white woman with a lifelong dietary calcium deficiency (Avioli, 1983). Blacks, who have a greater bone mass than whites at all ages, have a lower incidence of symptomatic osteoporosis. In the Caucasian population, the incidence of symptomatic disease is lower in persons from southern Europe and the Mediterranean basin than in those of northern European extraction. Racial differences in incidence may reflect differences in peak bone mass rather than rates of bone loss, which are quite constant in all ethnic groups (Kleere-koper, Tolia, & Parfitt, 1981).

Nutrition

Adequate calcium intake is as vital in maintaining peak bone mass as in attaining it. The body regulates few parameters with greater fidelity than the concentration of ionized calcium in the blood. Extracellular ionized calcium represents less than 1% of the body's calcium stores, but is the metabolically active fraction of the body's calcium and is critically important for numerous life-sustaining processes, including enzymatic reactions, mitochondrial function, cell membrane maintenance, intercellular communication, interneuronal transmission, neuromuscular transmission, muscular contraction, and blood clotting. An elaborate endocrine system maintains the serum ionized calcium concentration within a very narrow physiologic range. When this level falls, even momentarily, the body restores it to normal through its parathyroid hormone (PTH)-vitamin D system by effecting calcium absorption, reabsorption and resorption on the gastrointestinal, renal and skeletal endorgans, respectively (Heaney, Recker, & Saville, 1977; Parfitt, 1983). Despite popular beliefs, our need for calcium increases as we grow older. The National Research Council of the National Academy of Sciences has established recommended daily dietary allowances of calcium for all age groups. These values reflect the average amount of calcium needed to maintain positive calcium balance and prevent the body from drawing on the mineral stores banked in bone. For young adults, the recommended allowance is 800 mg daily. Unfortunately, large-scale dietary surveys of women with osteoporosis show that the average American woman consumes less than 500 mg of calcium daily (NIH Consensus, 1984).

Absorption of calcium from the upper gastrointestinal tract becomes less efficient with age; thus, older persons need more dietary calcium to maintain a positive calcium balance. Dairy products are the primary source of dietary calcium. An 8-oz. glass of skim milk provides approximately 250 mg of calcium. Healthy premenopausal women over age 30 may need as much as 1000 mg of calcium a day (the amount supplied by a quart of milk). In pregnant women or those over age 50, the recommended allowance increases to more than 1500 mg. Lactating women need 2 g of calcium daily to prevent untimely catabolism of bone (Avioli, 1983).

Calcium consumption may be inadequate in persons with heritable or acquired lactase deficiency. Since ingestion of dairy products can cause gastrointestinal discomfort in such persons, they avoid these foods.

Protein consumption also affects daily calcium requirements, as increased protein intake accelerates calcium excretion by the kidney. Doubling the daily protein intake increases urinary calcium losses by 50%, and the high-protein diet common in western industrialized countries may be a major cause of accelerated bone loss in these populations.

The vitamin D metabolite $1,25\text{-}(OH)_2D_3$ is the active hormone that helps maintain normal serum calcium and phosphate levels by increasing both absorption of these substances from the intestine and their resorption from bone. About half of our vitamin D_3 comes from dietary sources and the remainder from an endogenous reaction in the skin stimulated by ultraviolet radiation. Only a few natural foods, such as fish liver oils, contain vitamin D. Most milk sold in the United States is fortified with 400 IU of vitamin D per quart (Dairy Council, 1984). The elderly are frequently mildly vitamin D-deficient because of meager exposure to sunlight, decreased intake of milk and other dairy products, and decreased intestinal absorption of vitamin D. The recommended daily dietary allowance of vitamin D is 400 IU for young adults. For the elderly, 800 IU daily is recommended. Larger amounts are not advised routinely and may cause hypercalcemia.

Age and Sex

Once the skeleton has matured, skeletal mass remains relatively constant until the fifth decade, when it begins to decline. Bone mass decreases more rapidly in women than in men, and at locally variable rates throughout the skeleton. Average bone loss is approximately 0.5% a year after age 40.

Sex differences in bone loss are dramatic. At any given age, bone mass is greater in men than in women. Moreover, in the decade after age 40, men lose only about 0.5% to 0.75% of bone mass yearly, while women lose bone at more than twice that rate (1.5% to 2% a year). Following menopause, the rate of bone loss in some women may temporarily approach 3% a year (Avioli, 1977).

Endocrine Factors

In addition to age- and sex-related effects on bone loss, endocrine and metabolic changes influence the development of osteoporosis. In both osteoporotic and normal elderly women, vitamin D metabolite levels are normal. However, in elderly patients with osteoporosis, the kidney's production of $1,25\text{-}(OH)_2D_3$ in response to PTH infusion is impaired. Research supports the theory that deficient secretory reserves of $1,25\text{-}(OH)_2D_3$-whether secondary to age, gonadal steroid insufficiency, or other factors—may help explain older osteoporotic persons' inability to adapt to the calcium-poor diet common in this age group (Dairy Council, 1984; Francis, Peacock, Taylor, Storer, & Nordin, 1984; Slovik, Adams, Neer, Holick & Potts, 1982; Wallach, 1979). (See Figure 1.)

Causes of Osteoporosis

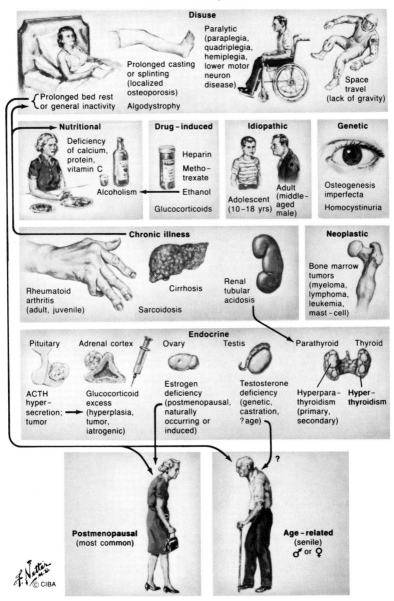

Physical Activity and Weight-Bearing Stress

Weight-bearing activity is essential to skeletal health. Mechanical weight-bearing stress is perhaps the most important exogenous factor affecting bone development and remodeling. A sedentary person is more likely to become osteoporotic than an active person who engages daily in some form of weight-bearing exercise. (See Figure 2.)

The marked reduction in gravitational field that results in the weightless environment of space flight leads to profound and rapid losses of skeletal and muscle mass despite vigorous physical activity (Avioli, 1983). More common causes of osteoporosis resulting from decreasing the muscular forces acting on bone include immobilization of a limb in a cast, splint or orthotic device; denervation of a peripheral nerve or of the spinal cord (e.g., paraplegia, quadriplegia or poliomyelitis); and prolonged bed rest.

Endocrine-Mediated Bone Loss

Endocrine abnormalities may cause osteoporosis and should be investigated in any young or middle-aged person with osteopenia. Numerous hormones affect skeletal remodeling and, hence, skeletal mass. In elderly patients, endocrine-mediated osteoporosis can occur in conjunction with postmenopausal or age-related osteoporosis. Only the most common endocrine disorders that can cause a loss of bone are considered in this discussion (Avioli, 1983; Wallach, 1979).

Hypogonadism causes bone loss in both men and women. All osteopenia seen in postmenopausal women has a hypogonadal component. Osteopenia will develop early following surgically induced menopause.

Hyperthyroidism, whether caused by glandular hyperactivity or secondary to overzealous replacement therapy in a patient with hypothyroidism, increases bone turnover and remodeling. Bone resorption exceeds bone formation, resulting in a net decrease in bone mass. Mild hyperthyroidism may escape clinical detection. Triiodothyronine resin uptake (T_3RU) and the thyroxine (T_4) levels should be determined when hyperthyroidism is suspected.

Hyperparathyroidism, either primary or secondary, also increases bone turnover and remodeling, causing a net increase in bone resorption. These conditions result in a fibrous proliferation of

Daily Exercises for Spinal Health

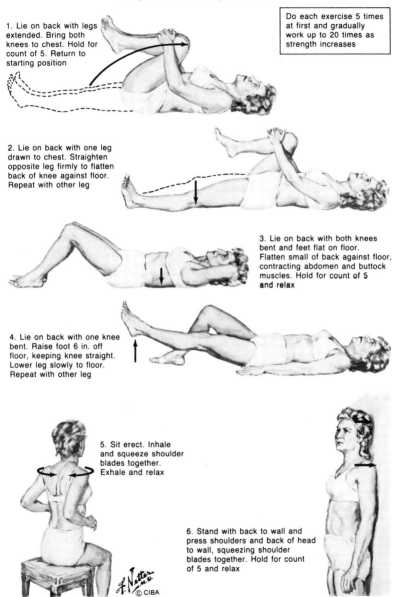

1. Lie on back with legs extended. Bring both knees to chest. Hold for count of 5. Return to starting position

Do each exercise 5 times at first and gradually work up to 20 times as strength increases

2. Lie on back with one leg drawn to chest. Straighten opposite leg firmly to flatten back of knee against floor. Repeat with other leg

3. Lie on back with both knees bent and feet flat on floor. Flatten small of back against floor, contracting abdomen and buttock muscles. Hold for count of 5 **and relax**

4. Lie on back with one knee bent. Raise foot 6 in. off floor, keeping knee straight. Lower leg slowly to floor. Repeat with other leg

5. Sit erect. Inhale and squeeze shoulder blades together. Exhale and relax

6. Stand with back to wall and press shoulders and back of head to wall, squeezing shoulder blades together. Hold for count of 5 and relax

FIGURE 2. © Copyright 1983, CIBA Pharmaceutical Company, Division of CIBA-GEIGY Corporation. Reprinted with permission from *Clinical Symposia* illustrated by Frank Netter, MD. All rights reserved.

the bone marrow (osteitis fibrosa cystica). Primary glandular hyperactivity can be associated with bone pain, pseudogout, peptic ulcer, constipation, nephrolithiasis, fatigue, thirst, pancreatitis and central nervous system disturbances, all resulting from the hypercalcemic effect of increased PTH secretion. However, in many persons the glandular disturbance is mild and not associated with the secondary conditions listed. Hyperparathyroidism should be suspected whenever several of the conditions mentioned are present in an osteopenic person and whenever hypercalcemia and hyupophosphatemia are discovered incidentally on routine blood chemistry determinations.

Hyperadrenalism, or chronic glucocorticoid excess, whether endogenous (Cushing's syndrome) or iatrogenic, leads to a refractory state of decreased bone mass. Chronic glucocorticoid excess reduces bone mineral and connective tissue metabolism. Because of their atrophic effect on the lining cells of the jejunum, glucocorticoids decrease intestinal absorption of calcium. In addition to this indirect catabolic effect on both osteoid and bone mineral, glucocorticoids exert a direct antianabolic effect on bone metabolism (Baylink, 1983).

The combined direct and indirect effects of glucocorticoids cause a decrease in bone mass, which results in osteoporosis. Symptoms are usually more severe in the axial skeleton than in the appendicular skeleton because of the larger surface area and increased rate of bone turnover in axial trabecular bone. Despite some promising reports, in general, glucocorticoid-induced osteopenia remains difficult to treat. However, the rate of bone loss may be decreased by appropriate dietary calcium supplementation.

Diet-Related Bone Loss

Chronic alcoholism is the most common cause of bone loss in young men and is related to the typically poor diet of chronic alcoholics. In addition, ethanol had been implicated as a cause of decreased intestinal calcium absorption. Skeletal mass in alcoholics is less than that in age- and sex-matched controls.

Disease-Related Bone Loss

Chronic illness of almost any kind can lead to osteopenia, with malnutrition and disuse the major contributing factors. Osteopenia is also a common complication of most bone marrow tumors. Multiple myeloma, the most common primary bone tumor in adults, may be associated with profound generalized axial and appendicular osteopenia. Myeloma cells produce a circulating osteoclast-activating factor that is a potent stimulator of bone resorption. Myeloma should be suspected in any adult over age 50 who has symptomatic osteopenia. Anemia, proteinuria, and a sedimentation rate greater than 100 mm/h suggest the diagnosis. Serum protein electrophoresis should be done when multiple myeloma is suspected. If results are inconclusive, urinary immunoelectrophoresis should be done. Approximately 1% of myelomas are nonsecretory, and a definitive diagnosis in all patients is made by bone marrow biopsy. Studies have shown that about 1% of patients who have symptomatic osteoporosis have multiple myeloma. Leukemia, lymphoma, and the extremely rare mast-cell tumor also may be associated with osteoporosis (Avioli, 1977).

DIAGNOSIS OF OSTEOPOROSIS

If hypertension is a silent killer, osteoporosis is a silent thief. It insidiously robs the skeleton of its banked resources, often for decades, before the bone is weak enough to sustain a spontaneous fracture. Although the entire skeleton may be susceptible to age-related and postmenopausal bone loss, regions of high trabecular bone remodeling, such as the thoracic and lumbar vertebral bodies, ribs, proximal femur and humerus, and distal radius sustain the most damage. Gross morphologic changes seen with osteoporosis include increased porosity of both trabecular and cortical bone. Characteristic changes seen in the long bones include increased intracortical porosity, as well as enlargement of the medullary cavities caused by a net increase of endosteal bone resorption over periosteal new bone formation.

Early Symptoms

An episode of acute pain in the middle to low thoracic or high lumbar regions while at rest or during routine daily activity such as standing, bending, or lifting may be the earliest symptom of osteoporosis. The episode is often precipitated by routine activity that under normal circumstances would not be stressful enough to cause a fracture. The onset of pain is sudden. Spinal movement is severely restricted. Pain intensifies with sitting or standing and is relieved considerably with bed rest in the fully recumbent position. Coughing, sneezing, and straining to move the bowels can cause excruciating exacerbation of the pain. Loss of appetite, abdominal distention, and ileus secondary to retroperitoneal hemorrhage may accompany lower thoracic and upper lumbar compression fractures. Some persons who sustain a compression fracture in the midthoracic spine are relatively symptom-free except for slight discomfort along the costal margins, incremental loss in height, and mild thoracic kyphosis (Frost, 1981).

Appendicular Fractures

The most common clinical symptom of osteoporosis is back pain secondary to vertebral compression fracture. However, in some persons, a fracture of the proximal femur sustained after little or no trauma or a fracture of the distal radius sustained during a fall on the outstretched wrist is the first indication of the disease. The incidence of fractures of the proximal femur increases with age, and shows a bimodal peak. Intracapsular fractures of the femur occur most commonly between ages 65 and 75, while the incidence of intertrochanteric fractures peaks nearly 10 years later between ages 75 and 85. Numerous explanations for this bimodal distribution have been postulated, but the true reasons remain unclear.

Work-up in Symptomatic Disease

Although postmenopausal osteoporosis is the most common form of symptomatic bone loss seen in clinical practice, other causes must often be systematically excluded. The history may suggest bone loss secondary to hyperthyroidism (primary and iatrogenic), primary hyperparathyroidism, hypercortisolism, myeloma or osteomalacia. An exhaustive history is therefore essential in making the differential diagnosis. After the history is taken, a complete physical examination is done, and standing anteroposterior and lateral radiographs of the thoracic and lumbar spine are obtained (Avioli, 1983).

An extensive history facilitates selection of appropriate baseline tests. In uncomplicated postmenopausal disease, results of routine laboratory tests are normal and do not assess the extent or rate of bone loss or indicate the prognosis. Even in severe postmenopausal disease, serum calcium, inorganic phosphorus, and alkaline phosphatase levels are usually within the normal range, although alkaline phosphatase levels may rise after a fracture.

Osteomalacia, also known as adult rickets, must be considered in the differential diagnosis of osteopenia. Osteomalacia should be suspected in a patient with generalized myopathy, bone pain and tenderness, and symmetrical long-bone fractures. Abnormalities in vitamin D absorption and metabolism often play a major role in the pathogenesis of the disease. The diagnosis is confirmed by fluorescent microscopic examination of undecalcified trabecular bone tissue taken by transiliac bone biopsy after time-separated double-tetracycline labeling. Levels of 25-(OH)D$_3$ and 1,25-(OH)$_2$D$_3$ must also be ascertained when osteomalacia is suggested.

Finally, in centers where the diagnostic techniques are available, noninvasive tests to monitor the progression of bone loss and the response to treatment may be desirable. These include quantitative assessments of bone mineral content and density. The technetium 99m methylene diphosphonate bone scan is useful in documenting new compression fractures in persons with preexisting severe vertebral collapse.

Clinical Findings

In the early stages following an acute thoracic compression fracture, physical examination reveals the patient to be in marked discomfort while sitting or standing. Spinal movement is considerably reduced, with more restriction in flexion than in extension. Previous anterior compression fractures may have caused thoracic kyphosis (dowager's hump). The lumbar spine may be involved, with progressive loss in lumbar lordosis. Axial height may be decreased. A discrepancy is noted between the standing height and arm span (as measured from the tip of the middle finger across the chest to the tip of the contralateral middle finger). Normally these measurements are equal, but with recurrent episodes of vertebral collapse, the height decreases and the difference between the arm span and the standing height increases.

Paravertebral muscle spasms are palpable and often visible. The spine is tender to deep palpation and to percussion over the fracture, but bony point tenderness is usually absent because the fracture is in the anterior vertebral body rather than in the palpable posterior spinal elements.

The acute episode does not usually alter the neurologic findings of previous examinations. Spontaneous vertebral compression fractures are stable injuries, although appendicular radiculopathies are common with thoracic or upper lumbar compression fractures and cause either unilateral or bilateral pain radiating anteriorly along the costal margin of the affected nerve root. Spinal cord or cauda equina involvement suggests other conditions such as infection or tumor, Paget's disease, metastatic disease, myeloma or lymphoma. During the intervals (often years) between compression fractures, most patients are totally pain-free. However, some continue to be plagued with chronic, dull, aching, postural pain in the midthoracic and upper lumbar region that responds symptomatically to frequent, intermittent horizontal rest.

With each episode of segmental vertebral collapse and progressive kyphosis, the patient's height may decrease 2 to 4 cm. In 95% of postmenopausal patients with symptomatic osteoporosis, more than six radiographically evident vertebral fractures occur over a period of approximately 10 years. Seventy-five percent of patients lose at least 10 cm in height. Once the spine has collapsed to the point where the lower ribs come to rest on the iliac crest, further significant loss in height is not likely, although loss of bone mass may continue.

Two of the clinically disturbing, long-term side effects of progressive vertebral compression fractures occur as a result of the decrease in size of the thoracic and abdominal cavities. The patient becomes aware of diminished exercise tolerance as a result of disease-related postural changes. Early satiety is noted, with abdominal protrusion secondary to severe lumbar vertebral collapse. The patient feels bloated after ingesting small amounts of food. Circumferential pachydermal skin folds develop at the rib and pelvic margins as the disease progresses.

Radiographic findings. Standing anteroposterior and lateral radiographs of the thoracic and lumbar spine should be obtained in any patient suspected of having a compression fracture (Frost, 1981).

Measurements of bone mass. Although plain radiographs are useful in the initial evaluation of osteopenia, they are the least accurate, least precise method of assessing bone density. During the past decade, noninvasive radiographic and radioisotope techniques have been developed to determine skeletal mass. These techniques (Quantitative Computed Tomographic Scanning of Lumbar vertebral bodies and Dual Photon absorptiometry of the Lumbar spine) are precise, sensitive and safe. Actual quantitation of bone mass in vivo helps to establish the severity of bone loss in an osteopenic patient and serves as a baseline for evaluation of therapy (Cohn, 1982).

Transiliac bone biopsy. Several important advances in the last 20 years have made transiliac bone biopsy a useful diagnostic tool in evaluating metabolic bone diseases and disorders of skeletal homeostasis (Frost, 1969; Lane & Vigorita, 1983). Bone biopsy is not recommended for every woman with postmenopausal disease. However, biopsy is an important diagnostic tool in patients less than age 50 who have symptomatic or incidentally discovered asymptomatic osteopenia and in any patient, even an elderly postmenopausal patient, in whom osteomalacia is suspected. Because of the inherent problem of regional sampling error, bone biopsy should not be used to establish a diagnosis of osteoporosis; rather, it should be used to exclude a diagnosis of osteomalacia.

MANAGEMENT

The management of osteoporosis has two facets: (1) treatment of symptomatic disease and its sequelae and (2) maintenance of skeletal mass and integrity.

Treatment of Acute Symptoms

Spinal compression fractures can be extremely painful and cause significant short-term morbidity. However, even in a severely osteopenic skeleton, the fracture heals quickly, regardless of treatment. Thus, the goals of therapy are to relieve pain, provide comfortable mechanical support for the spine, arrange assistance in activities of daily living, coordinate a rehabilitation program, and provide encouragement and reassurance to the patient and family.

Following an acute spinal compression fracture, the patient is most comfortable in a supine position so that the spine is free of excessive mechanical stress. The patient should stay in bed, in a horizontal position, with no more than a small pillow beneath the head until the acute pain begins to subside (7 to 14 days). Although patients are initially most comfortable at complete bed rest, most prefer to use the bathroom or a bedside commode rather than a bedpan.

Despite the detrimental effect on the skeleton, the period of bed rest is often necessary for the patient's comfort. A firm mattress prevents spinal flexion, which may aggravate the traumatic kyphosis, and a pillow under the knees relieves excessive stress on the lower back. A sheepskin mattress cover improves skin care and reduces the risk of pressure sores over prominent spinous processes. Short-term oral administration of narcotic analgesics is recommended. Rarely, a patient may need stronger narcotics given parenterally. Special care must be taken to avoid constipation, urinary retention, and respiratory depression in elderly patients taking these medications. When necessary, stool softeners and laxatives should be given to prevent fecal impaction. Short-term use of mild muscle relaxants diminishes the paravertebral muscle spasms that accompany fracture.

Support services during the period of acute infirmity must be tailored to the individual patient. For most patients, a family member or a visiting nurse can provide assistance, but when a patient lives alone or cannot call on family, a short hospitalization may be necessary.

Once the acute pain begins to subside and the patient can turn in bed more comfortably, mobilization should begin. The patient should attempt to sit or stand for periods of not longer than 10 to 15 minutes several times a day. Since sitting and standing exert similar forces on the vertebral body, the patient may choose the most comfortable position. As pain subsides, the patient should increase the frequency and duration of mobilization periods. More rapid mobilization is not likely to impede healing or to cause further structural harm, but may prolong the period of discomfort.

For severe pain following compression fracture in the middle to lower thoracic regions, a rigid thoracolumbar hyperextension orthosis provides external support, alleviates flexion forces on the affected vertebral segments, and allows easier mobilization. Some patients find the rigid device too restricting and prefer a three-point semirigid thoracolumbar extension orthosis that discourages the kyphotic or stooped posture. Still other patients choose to forego orthotic devices altogether. These devices should be recommended on an individual basis, with consideration of the degree of discomfort the patient feels when sitting or standing. The patient should use the orthotic device when erect but need not wear it when in bed.

Other aids to mobilization include low-heeled, soft-soled shoes with foam or plastazote inserts that cushion the concussive forces transmitted to the spine during weight bearing. A cane may provide extra support and help the patient regain balance during the transition from complete bed rest to normal ambulation, and is especially important for the elderly person who may have problems with proprioception.

Instruction in proper back care is an essential component of the rehabilitative process. Patients should be shown how to avoid unnecessary spinal compression forces in lifting and bending. They should avoid movable rugs and polished floors and take precautions to prevent falls, which result not only in spinal compression fractures, but also in hip, shoulder and forearm fractures. After 6 to 8 weeks, most patients are relatively pain-free and can resume prefracture activity levels although a fear of more fractures is often the most limiting factor. Patients who continue to have back pain after periods of activity may benefit from short periods of intermittent bed rest, 15 to 20 minutes several times each day.

MAINTENANCE OF SKELETAL MASS

Oral Calcium Supplementation

Inadequate calcium intake is common in the elderly. The incidence of hip fractures is lower in women with adequate calcium intake than in those with inadequate intake. Low-sodium diets—often desirable in treatment of hypertension—are also low in calcium and may need to be supplemented.

Hypercalcemia, hypercalciuria, and renal stone formation are rare in uncomplicated postmenopausal osteoporosis. However, all patients receiving dietary calcium supplements should be encouraged to maintain a high urine volume. Before supplementation is started in a patient in whom hypercalciuria is suspected or who has a history of nephrolithiasis or urolithiasis, a 24-hour urine collection to assess calcium, phosphorus, and creatinine levels should be done. Prolonged bed rest or immobilization, sarcoidosis, metastatic malignancy, multiple myeloma, primary hyperparathyroidism, idiopathic hypercalciuria, hypervitaminosis D, or thiazide diuretic therapy can cause either transient or more prolonged hypercalcemia. After these and related conditions are ruled out, dietary calcium supplementation can be administered with relative impunity.

Patients should eat foods high in calcium (e.g., dairy products, sardines, and green leafy vegetables). The average postmenopausal woman requires the equivalent of six 8-oz. glasses of skim milk daily. Nonprescription oral calcium supplements, such as calcium carbonate, phosphate, lactate or gluconate, can supplement a calcium-poor diet. The carbonate preparation has the highest percentage of calcium, containing 40% elemental calcium by weight; calcium phosphate contains 31%, calcium lactate 13%, and calcium gluconate only 9%. Patient compliance is greatest with the carbonate preparation, because fewer tablets are needed to achieve recommended calcium intake. However, the carbonate preparation can cause bloating and flatulence, and some patients prefer calcium lactate or gluconate (Avioli, 1977; Avioli, 1983; Frost, 1981; Heaney, Recker & Saville, 1977; Heaney, Recker, & Saville, 1978; NIH, 1984). (See Figure 3.)

Vitamin D therapy. Daily exposure to sunshine is recommended. Vitamin D supplementation within recommended guidelines is essential in persons deficient in this vitamin. However, it should be emphasized that treatment of postmenopausal osteoporosis with massive doses of vitamin D (50,000 IU twice weekly) can lead to dangerous hypercalcemia and is no longer recommended.

Estrogen replacement therapy. Estrogen therapy following the menopause inhibits bone resorption and helps preserve both axial and appendicular bone mass (Christiansen, Christensen, Larsen & Transbol, 1982). Estrogen therapy is most effective in the perimenopausal period, before bone loss becomes severe, and may be indicated to prevent untimely bone loss in women in whom menopause is surgically induced. Dosages of less than 0.6 mg daily are not as effective in preventing trabecular bone loss from the axial skeleton. The slightly increased risk of endometrial cancer with estrogen therapy must be considered. Patients taking estrogens must have close gynecologic follow-up care (Christiansen, Christensen, Larsen & Transbol, 1982; Recker, Saville, & Heaney, 1977).

Exercise. As previously discussed, regular weight-bearing activity is essential for the maintenance of bone mass. The minimum amount of weight bearing necessary to maintain constant bone mass throughout adult life has not been determined. However, a daily program of weight-bearing activity, including a 30-minute walk (which has the added benefit of exposing the face and hands to sunlight, a stimulus of vitamin D formation in the skin), is recommended (Korcok, 1982).

Sodium flouride therapy. The discovery that osteoporosis is less prevalent in some areas where fluoride intake is high, coupled with

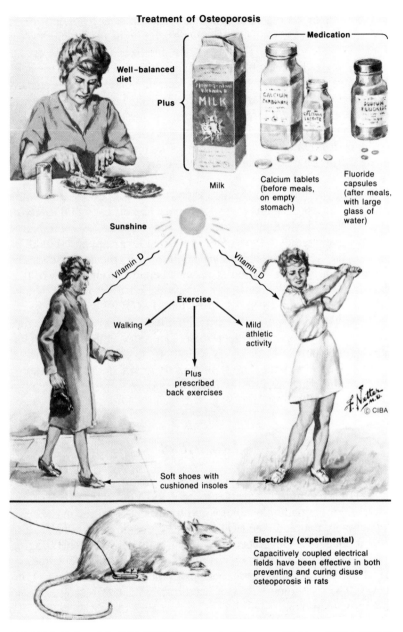

Treatment of Osteoporosis

FIGURE 3. © Copyright 1983, CIBA Pharmaceutical Company, Division of CIBA-GEIGY Corporation. Reprinted with permission from *Clinical Symposia* illustrated by Frank Netter, MD. All rights reserved.

the finding of increased density in fluorotic bone, has led to the speculation that fluorides may be beneficial in the treatment of some forms of osteoporosis. Fluoride both stabilizes the mineral crystal and stimulates the osteoblast to form new matrix. Although the newly synthesized and radiographically denser bone is not structurally or materially normal, early evidence showing a decreased incidence of vertebral body compression fractures in patients taking fluorides, as compared with untreated controls, suggests that the bone may be stronger following fluoride therapy. Calcium intake must be adequate during fluoride treatment to avoid an osteomalacia-like condition with brittle bones.

Despite publicity about the osteotrophic properties of sodium fluoride, its use remains investigational. The efficacy and safety of sodium fluoride therapy are currently being assessed in several large prospective studies. Two other investigational agents should be mentioned. The peptide hormone calcitonin and the anabolic steroid stanozolol are being studied at various centers around the world to determine their effectiveness in inhibiting bone resorption (Riggs, Seeman, Hodgson, Taves, & O'Fallon, 1982).

Prophylactic therapy. Women who are at increased risk of symptomatic postmenopausal osteoporosis can reduce that risk by maintaining adequate calcium levels with diet and calcium supplements, taking estrogen in the perimenopausal period under gynecologic supervision, and engaging regularly in outdoor weight-bearing exercise (Aloia, 1981; NIH, 1984).

FRONTIERS

Our knowledge of osteoporosis is far from complete, and the underlying mechanisms are yet to be discovered. Nevertheless, research into the pathophysiology and treatment is promising. Use of capacitively coupled electrical fields to prevent osteoporosis and to treat it once it has developed is being investigated, with encouraging results. This novel approach is a direct extension of work with electrical fields to stimulate osteogenesis in the healing of fracture nonunion. The technique has been used to treat disuse osteoporosis in laboratory animals.

The endemic problems of osteoporosis pose major challenges to the medical community. We must increase public awareness of the importance of adequate calcium intake and weight-bearing activity throughout life; continue our development of safe, noninvasive, inexpensive methods of assessing bone mass in vivo; identify patients at high risk before symptoms develop; expand research in the cellular biology of aging in musculoskeletal tissues; and investigate, through prospective studies, biologic and pharmacologic agents that can retard bone loss, stimulate new bone formation, and selectively uncouple the process in favor of bone formation.

REFERENCES

Aloia, J.F. (1981). Exercise and skeletal health. *Journal of the American Geriatric Society,* 29, 104-107.

Avioli, L.V. (1977). Osteoporosis: Pathogenesis and therapy. In L.V. Avioli & S.M. Krane, (Eds.), *Metabolic bone disease* (pp. 307-384). New York: Academic Press.

Avioli, L.V. (Ed.). (1983). *The osteoporotic syndrome: Detection, prevention, and treatment.* New York: Grune & Stratton.

Baylink, D.J. (1983). Glucocorticoid-induced osteoporosis (editorial). *New England Journal of Medicine, 309,* 306-308.

Christiansen, C., Christensen, M.S., Larsen, N.E., & Transbol, I. (1982). Pathophysiological mechanisms of estrogen effect on bone metabolism. Dose-response relationships in early postmenopausal women. *Journal of Clinical Endocrinology and Metabolism, 55,* 1124-1130.

Cohn, S.H. (1982). Techniques for determining the efficacy of treatment of osteoporosis. *Calcified Tissue International, 34,* 433-438.

Dairy Council Digest. (1984). *55*(1), 1-8.

Francis, R.M., Peacock, M., Taylor, G.A., Storer, J.H. & Nordin, B.E. (1984). Calcium malabsorption in elderly women with vertebral fractures: Evidence for resistance to the action of vitamin D metabolites on the bowel. *Clinical Science, 66*(1), 103-107.

Frost, H.M. (1969). Tetracycline-based histological analysis of bone remodeling. *Calcified Tissue Research, 3,* 211-217.

Frost, H.M. (1981). Clinical management of the symptomatic osteoporotic patient. *Orthopaedic Clinics of North America, 12*(3), 671-681.

Garraway, W.M., Stauffer, R.M., Kurland, L.T., & O'Fallon, W.M. (1979). Limb fractures in a defined population. *Mayo Clinic Proceedings, 54,* 701-713.

Heaney, R.P., Recker, R.R., & Saville, P.D. (1977). Calcium balance and calcium requirements in middle-aged women. *American Journal of Clinical Nutrition, 30*(10), 1603-1611.

Heaney, R.P., Recker, R.R., & Saville, P.D. (1978). Menopausal changes in calcium balance performance. *Journal of Laboratory & Clinical Medicine, 92*(6), 953-963.

Ivey, J.L., & Baylink, D.J. (1981). Postmenopausal osteoporosis: Proposed roles of defective coupling and estrogen deficiency. *Metabolic Bone Disease & Related Research, 3,* 3-7.

Kelsey, J.L., White, A.A., Pastides, H., & Bisbee, G.E. (1979). The impact of musculoskeletal disorders on the population of the United States. *Journal of Bone & Joint Surgery, 61-A,* 959-964.

Kleerekoper, M.B., Tolia, K., & Parfitt, A.M. (1981). Nutritional, endocrine and demographic aspect of osteoporosis. *Orthopaedic Clinics of North America, 12,* 547-558.

Korcok, M. (1982). Add exercise to calcium in osteoporosis prevention. *Journal of The American Medical Association, 247,* 1106-1112.

Lane, J.M., & Vigorita, V.J. (1983). Osteoporosis. *Journal of Bone Joint & Surgery, 65-A,* 274-278.

National Institutes of Health Consensus Development Conference Statement on Osteoporosis–Draft–April 2-4, 1984.

Parfitt, A.M. (1983). Dietary risk factors for age-related bone loss and fractures. *Lancet, 8360,* 1181-1185.

Recker, R.R., Saville, P.D., & Heaney, R.P. (1977). Effect of estrogens and calcium carbonate on bone loss in postmenopausal women. *Annals of Internal Medicine, 87*(6), 649-655.

Riggs, B.L., Seeman, E., Hodgson, S.F., Taves, D.R., & O'Fallon, W.M. (1982). Effect of the flouride/calcium regimen on vertebral fracture occurrence in postmenopausal osteoporosis. Comparison with conventional therapy. *New England Journal of Medicine, 306,* 446-450.

Slovik, D.M., Adams, J.S., Neer, R.M., Holick, M.F., & Potts, J.T. (1982). Deficient production of 1,25-dihydroxy-vitamin-D in elderly osteoporotic patients. *New England Journal of Medicine, 305,* 372-374.

Wallach, S. (1979) Hormonal factors in osteoporosis. *Clinical Orthopaedics & Related Research, 144,* 284-292.

Whyte, M.P., Bergfeld, M.A., Murphy, W.A., Avioli, L.V., & Teitelbaum, S.V. (1982). Postmenopausal osteoporosis. A heterogeneous disorder as assessed by histomorphometric analysis of iliac crest bone from untreated patients. *American Journal of Medicine, 72*(2), 193-202.

Psychological Aspects
of Aging in Women

Jane Porcino, PhD

ABSTRACT. Older women are forced to cope with many societal myths and negative stereotypes. This paper reviews the influence of these stereotypes as well as some of the other psychological concerns of women who are aging. Losses such as widowhood and divorce as well as the problem of loneliness are discussed.

The autumn of a woman's life is far richer than the spring if only she becomes aware in time, and harvests the ripening fruit before it falls and rots and is trampled underfoot. The winter which follows is not barren if the harvest has been stored. (Castillejo, 1973)

These words written by an elderly woman psychologist speak in a poetic way of the necessary tasks that women need to perform in order to cope with the last transition of the life cycle, old age. This paper will discuss the sociological and psychological concerns of older women: the double standard, personal losses, sexuality and intimacy, and how women cope with the aging process.

When we talk about aging we are primarily talking about women, for females make up almost 60% of the aging population. There are 16.6 million women over the age of 65 in America today, as compared to 10.7 million men. In 1900, men outnumbered women in the 65+ years. By 1930, we had equal numbers of each sex in this age group. Today there are approximately 150 women over the age of 65, to every 100 men (at age 85+ those numbers are 220 to 100). White women can expect to live 8 years longer than their male counterparts; black women 9 years longer. This disparity is likely to continue to widen (Statistical Bulletin, 1984). Old age is clearly a

---

Dr. Porcino is the author of *Growing Older, Getting Better: A Handbook for Women in the Second Half of Life* published in 1983.

115

territory more traveled by women (Markson, 1983). These are the statistics, but what are the social, psychological and economic implications of this 20th century change in the sex ratio of our aging population?

THE DOUBLE STANDARD OF AGING

To begin with, the double standard of aging forms the basis for the stereotypical view of today's older woman as dependent, passive, incompetent, and unattractive. Increasing age is perceived more negatively for women than for men (Datan & Lohmann, 1980). Changes in physical attractiveness (whether real or viewed as such by society), affect the mental health of older women (Block, Davidson & Grambs, 1981). "Women have a more intimate relation to aging than men do, simply because one of the accepted 'women's' occupations is taking pains to keep one's face and body from showing the signs of growing older" (Sontag, 1979). Sontag contends that beauty is women's business and this concept enslaves them with the notion that they must look young. Despite today's many beautiful older women, society's standard for beauty is still youth (Sontag, 1979).

SEXUALITY

Older women who are suddenly single through widowhood or divorce, and who are trying to attract men, are the most worried about their appearance. Aging women are often dismissed as desirable sex partners (Abu-Laban, 1981), despite the fact that research indicates a healthy older woman, with a responsive partner, will find her sex drive remains fairly constant well into advanced age. The studies of Masters and Johnson (1966) assert optimistically that there is no time limit drawn by advancing years to female sexuality. Earlier, Kinsey, Pomeroy, Martin and Gebhard (1955) established that a woman of 80 had the same capacity for orgasm as she had in her early twenties. Baruch, Barnett and Rivers, in their three-year study of mid-life women, reported in "Lifeprints" (1983) that the women of their sample showed no decline in sexual satisfaction as they aged—with many reporting a steady growth in their sexual interest and responsiveness with aging. However, there are currently real limitations in expressing this sexuality for older women (Abu-Laban, 1981). These limitations are socialization, widowhood, divorce, the unlikelihood of remarriage, and social pressure. The most outstanding factor here is the lack of a partner. Two-thirds of all women over age 65 are single in contrast with only one-fourth of their male peers. The average age of widowhood is 56. The increasing rate of divorce in marriages of more than 30 years duration, has even produced a new descriptive term, "the graying divorcee." Men who are widowed and divorced in their later years quickly remarry, usually to much younger women—leaving three-quarters of all men over 65 married, as compared to one-third of all like-aged women. Since women tend to marry older men, and live longer in our society, there are few men available as intimates in old age.

WIDOWHOOD, DIVORCE AND LONELINESS

Indeed, the life event which has the greatest impact on a woman's life may well be the death of her spouse, followed closely by divorce (Holmes & Rahe, 1967). A surviving older widow or divorcee faces emotional as well as social problems associated with the loss of her mate. We live in a couple-oriented society in which a woman alone, and old, is in a very vulnerable position. Losing her spouse, a woman loses her lover, companion, someone who validates her, an escort for public events, a mate in couple interaction, someone to share household chores, her lifestyle, and often her married friends. The adjustment from being part of a pair to being alone causes a personal crisis of great import (Block, Davidson & Grambs, 1981).

The group of older single women most vulnerable to stress, are those who were dependent on their husband for economic support. Marital disruption is the major cause of the poverty of older women. Becoming suddenly single, all too often means becoming suddenly poor. Older women are 80% of the elderly poor, with a median annual income of $4,757 (U.S. Bureau of the Census, 1980). A widow's income can suddenly drop by as much as 42% (Porcino, 1983).

The ultimate task for the older widow or divorcee is to reconstruct her life. This is not easy, for grief produces loneliness (Lopata, Heinemann & Baum, 1982). "These feelings of loneliness, which may be intense enough to make a woman feel she is 'going crazy,' losing touch with reality, often lead to a transient depression characterized by apathy, withdrawal, and inactivity'' (Porcino, 1983). A support system is crucial at this time, and can be either informal or formal. Family and friends make up informal networks with the formal consisting of churches, voluntary associates, self-help groups, and activities outside the home (Lopata et al., 1982). As a strategy for coping with widowhood, Lopata et al. (1982) stress the ''self'' as a major resource, used in conjunction with family and friends. Grief work must be accomplished, leading most older women to a period of growth. Lowenthal and Robinson (1976) cite Blau's 1961 study which states that women have ''a certain flexibility in the object of close relationships, in this instance a shift after widowhood from the intimacy of marriage to that of same sex friendship.'' Late-life singlehood can be a positive turning point in a woman's life. Perhaps for the first time she can discover herself as a free, independent person, with her own right to personal space (Peplau, Bikson, Rook & Goodchilds, 1982).

Despite what they have in common, women who are suddenly single are not a homogeneous group. Widows seem less ego-damaged by their experience than older women who have been divorced after long-term marriages. The graying divorcee often has a shattered ego along with feelings of failure and intense anger (Porcino, 1983). She needs reassurance that she still has the capacity to make and sustain new relationships, to develop her own new social network. Today's no-fault divorce laws have often been a disaster for older women, who lose not only their spouse, but their home, health, insurance, and source of income. Alimony (or maintenance) may be limited to 3 to 5 years, ''just enough for a woman to get back on her feet.'' In our ageist society only a small number of older women are able to gain new skills and well-paying jobs. Most older women left by their spouse feel betrayed and bitter, with a personal sense of guilt that they couldn't make their marriage work.

LONELINESS

Perhaps the major mental health problem for older women is loneliness. The shock of being alone for both divorcees and widows leads to at least a temporary state of loneliness. In ''Emerging Women,'' Rogers (1980) describes two forms of loneliness: (1) separation and loss, death, divorce, rejection, and abandonment; (2)

being ignored or misunderstood by important others (this can happen within a marriage). She believes that in order to be truly in touch with ourselves, each of us needs to experience the state of loneliness. Loneliness has been defined as a deficit condition, an emotion of sadness caused by lack of meaningful contact with others (Peplan et al., 1982). Loneliness can kill: humans need the response of other living things. Without this sharing, a person can die of a broken heart (Lynch, 1976). In a moving short film called "Minnie Remembers" (Swanson, 1976), an older woman says:

How long has it been since someone touched me? 20 years? 20 years I've been a widow . . . respected, smiled at, but never touched, never held so close that loneliness was blotted out. Oh God . . . I'm so lonely."

These poignant words reflect one of our deepest fears about aging: loneliness.

ALCOHOLISM AND DRUG DEPENDENCY

Trying to find constructive answers to some of the losses in her later years, some older women turn to alcohol and drugs, and in severe cases, suicide (Anderson, 1979). Alcoholism is on the rise among older women (Limoges, 1981; Porcino, 1983). The breakup of marriages, changing lifestyles, and loneliness have caused many women to turn to alcohol in the years after 50. Older women are often closet-drinkers and therefore a conspiracy of silence may exist. Compounding the problem is the failure of doctors to recognize alcoholism among their older female patients. Diagnosis takes consideration and time, and often the symptoms of falling, malnutrition, and dementia are diagnosed as old age instead of alcoholism (Limoges, 1981). Fortunately many programs throughout the country are focusing in on the older female alcoholic, helping her develop a sense of self-esteem and a more positive attitude towards life. Success rates for women alcoholics are statistically higher than for men (Porcino, 1983).

Women in our society tend to be drug dependent. Elderly women use more legal medications than elderly men, and 50% of the nation's prescription drugs are prescribed to women over the age of 60

(Block et al., 1981). Drugs may be an escape from loneliness and physical pain. They are often "people substitutes" for lonely older women (Limoges, 1981). Psychopharmaceuticals, rather than psychotherapy and community resources, are all too often used with older women even though the aging female is quite receptive to therapy and counseling (Freeman, Sack & Berger, 1979).

COPING

One of a woman's strengths as she ages is her ability to remain connected to others and her continued capacity for intimacy. No matter what our age, we each need intimacy in our lives; at least one other person with whom we can share both pleasure and pain. We hunger for someone who will accept us as delightfully different, and that person can be female, male, young or old (Porcino, 1983). Perhaps one of our greatest challenges as we grow older is to thoughtfully and creatively search for intimacy, by trusting ourselves enough to take risks, and by exploring and experimenting with new and pleasurable living patterns and relationships. Although we have been socialized to seek only one significant other for an intimate relationship, perhaps as older women our search should be for a few intimate people to share our lives and to give us the physical comfort we need. *Lifeprints* (Baruch, Barnett & Rivers 1983) explores what makes an aging woman feel good about herself: being a valued member of society and in control of her life. The authors believe that women can achieve this positive self-image and enjoy their lives. Their research shows that the decline in an aging woman's self-esteem found in the early 1950s does not show up in the 1970s and 1980s. They argue that the women's movement has given women permission to expand their vision of self, at the same time that it has increased their opportunities. One of their major findings, dispelling a deeply rooted social myth, is that aging is more of a problem for women who remain at home than for women in the workforce. The happiest women in their study combined both working and family.

Older women are survivors in our society. They are learning how to cope with both the demands of their environment and their own personal needs; learning that they no longer have a restricted destiny; learning how to experience the moment and to take personal control over their own health and happiness. Ruth Jacobs (1979) advised older women to:

. . . nurture ourselves and others, cope with loss and re-engage, have friends and good leisure occupations, do meaningful and productive work as long as we are able . . . be eternally curious and learning seekers, be sufficiently narcissistic to respect and maintain the beauty of our bodies, doctor ourselves enough to think, dream and grow, and return to society with creativity and assertiveness to defend our own rights and those of others.

Chiriboga and Thurnher (1976) describe the older woman as finally "hitting her stride." She is assertive, capable of resolving her problems, confident and versatile. Today, we have thousands of older women role models who share with us lives full of new patterns of intimacy, hope, imagination, and accomplishments. Because of them, women in the second half of their lives are beginning to be recognized as a powerful force throughout the world.

REFERENCES

Abu-Laban (1981). Women and aging: A futurist perspective. *Psychology of Women Quarterly, 6* (1).

Anderson, B. (1979). *The aging game: Success and sex after 60.* New York: McGraw Hill.

Baruch, G., Barnett, R., & Rivers, C. (1983). *Lifeprints.* New York: McGraw Hill.

Block, M., Davidson, J., & Grambs, J. (1981). *Women over forty: Visions and realities.* New York: Springer.

Castillejo, I. (1973). *Knowing woman: A feminine psychology.* New York: Harper & Row.

Chiriboga, D., & Thurnher, M. (1976). Concept of self. In M. Lowenthal, & M. Thurnher (Eds.), *Four stages of life.* San Francisco: Jossey-Bass.

Datan, N. & Lohmann, N. (1980). *Transitions of aging.* New York: Academic Press.

Freeman, A., Sack, R., & Berger, P. (Eds.) 1979. *Psychiatry for the primary care physician.* Baltimore, Maryland: Williams & Wilkins.

Holmes, T. H., & Rahe, R. H. (1967). The social readjustment rating scale. *Journal of Psychomatic Research, 11.*

Jacobs, R. N. (1979). *Life after youth: Female, forty—What next?.* Boston: Beacon Press.

Kinsey, A., Pomeroy, W., Martin, C., & Gebhard, P. (1955). *Sexual behavior in the human female.* Philadelphia: Saunders.

Limoges, M. (1981). The older woman and alcohol abuse. In J. Bost (Ed.), *Social work and the elderly.* The University of Connecticut School of Social Work Career Training Program on Aging.

Lopata, H., Heinemann, G., & Baum, J. (1982). Loneliness Antecedents and coping strategies in the lives of widows. In L. A. Peplau & D. Perlman (Eds.), *Loneliness: A source book of current theory, research & therapy* (pp. 310-326). New York: Wiley.

Lowenthal, M., & Robinson, B. (1976). Social networks and isolation. In. R. H. Binstock & E. Shanus (Eds.), *Handbook of aging and the social sciences.* New York: Van Nostrand.

Lynch, J. (1976). *The broken heart: The medical consequences of loneliness in America.* New York: Basic Books.

Masters, W. & Johnson, V. (1966). *Human sexual response.* Boston: Little, Brown.

Markson, E. (1983). *Older women.* Lexington, Mass: Lexington Books.

Peplau, L. A., Bikson, T., Rook, K., & Goodchilds, J. (1982). Being old and living alone. In L. A. Peplau & D. Perlman (Eds.), *Loneliness: A sourcebook of current theory, research and therapy,* (pp. 327-350). New York: A. Wiley.

Porcino, J. (1983). *Growing older, getting better: A handbook for women in the second half of life.* Reading, Mass.: Addison-Wesley.

Rogers, N. (1980). *Emerging woman.* Point Reyes, Ca.: Personal Press.

Sontag, S. (1979). The double standard of aging. In J. H. Williams (Ed.), *Psychology of women: Selected readings,* (pp. 462-478). New York: Norton.

Statistical Bulletin. (1984, January-March). Metropolitan Life Insurance Co., Medical Department, Vol. 65, #1.

Swanson, D. (1976). *Minnie Remembers.* A film by Mass Media Ministries, Baltimore, Maryland.

U.S. Bureau of the Census. (1980, February). A statistical portrait of women in the United States. *Current population reports: Special studies.* Series P-23, #100, Washington, D.C.